Clinical OCT
Angiography Atlas

Clinical OCT Angiography Atlas

Editors

Bruno Lumbroso MD
Director, Centro Italiano Macula
Former Director, Rome Eye Hospital
Rome, Italy

David Huang MD PhD
Peterson Professor of Ophthalmology
Professor, Biomedical Engineering
Casey Eye Institute
Oregon Health and Science University
Portland, USA

Ching J Chen MD
Professor and Chairman
Director, Vitreoretinal Service
Department of Ophthalmology
University of Mississippi Medical Center
Mississippi, USA

Yali Jia PhD
Research Assistant Professor
Casey Eye Institute
Oregon Health and Science University
Portland, USA

Marco Rispoli MD
Staff Ophthalmologist, Department of Ophthalmology
Ospedale Nuova Regina Margherita
Centro Italiano Macula
Rome, Italy

André Romano MD
Department Ophthalmology
Federal University Sao Paulo
Voluntary Adjunct Professor
University of Miami, Miller School of Medicine
Director Neovista Eye Center
Americana, Brazil

Nadia K Waheed MD MPH
Assistant Professor in Ophthalmology
Tufts University School of Medicine
Boston, MA, USA

Foreword
James G Fujimoto

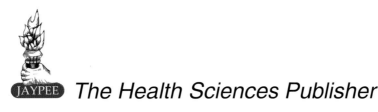

JAYPEE *The Health Sciences Publisher*

New Delhi | London | Philadelphia | Panama

Jaypee Brothers Medical Publishers (P) Ltd

Headquarters

Jaypee Brothers Medical Publishers (P) Ltd
4838/24, Ansari Road, Daryaganj
New Delhi 110 002, India
Phone: +91-11-43574357
Fax: +91-11-43574314
Email: jaypee@jaypeebrothers.com

Overseas Offices

J.P. Medical Ltd
83 Victoria Street, London
SW1H 0HW (UK)
Phone: +44 20 3170 8910
Fax: +44 (0)20 3008 6180
Email: info@jpmedpub.com

Jaypee Medical Inc
The Bourse
111 South Independence Mall East
Suite 835, Philadelphia, PA 19106, USA
Phone: +1 267-519-9789
Email: jpmed.us@gmail.com

Jaypee Brothers Medical Publishers (P) Ltd
Bhotahity, Kathmandu, Nepal
Phone: +977-9741283608
Email: kathmandu@jaypeebrothers.com

Jaypee-Highlights Medical Publishers Inc
City of Knowledge, Bld. 237, Clayton
Panama City, Panama
Phone: +1 507-301-0496
Fax: +1 507-301-0499
Email: cservice@jphmedical.com

Jaypee Brothers Medical Publishers (P) Ltd
17/1-B Babar Road, Block-B, Shaymali
Mohammadpur, Dhaka-1207
Bangladesh
Mobile: +08801912003485
Email: jaypeedhaka@gmail.com

Website: www.jaypeebrothers.com
Website: www.jaypeedigital.com

Clinical OCT Angiography Atlas

First Edition: **2015**
ISBN 978-93-5152-899-9
Printed at Replika Press Pvt. Ltd.

Contributors

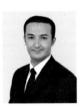

Adil El Maftouhi OD
Centre Rabelais, Lyon
Centre Explore Vision
XV XX Hospital, Service du Pr C BAUDOUIN
Paris, France

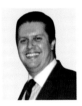

André Romano MD
Department Ophthalmology
Federal University Sao Paulo
Voluntary Adjunct Professor
University of Miami
Miller School of Medicine
Director Neovista Eye Center
Americana, Brazil

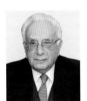

Bruno Lumbroso MD
Director, Centro Italiano Macula
Former Director, Rome Eye Hospital
Rome, Italy

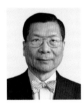

Ching J Chen MD
Professor and Chairman
Director of Vitreoretinal Service
Department of Ophthalmology
University of Mississippi Medical Center
Mississippi, USA

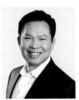

David Huang MD PhD
Peterson Professor of Ophthalmology
Professor of Biomedical Engineering
Casey Eye Institute
Oregon Health and Science University
Portland, USA

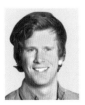

Eric M Moult PhD
Department of Electrical Engineering and
Research Laboratory of Electronics
Massachusetts Institute of Technology, and
Harvard MIT Department of Health Science and
Technology
Cambridge, MA, USA

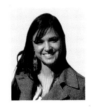

Gilda Cennamo MD PhD
Eye Clinic, Federico II University
Naples, Italy

James G Fujimoto PhD
Elihu Thomson Professor
Electrical Engineering and Computer Science
Massachusetts Institute of Technology
Cambridge, MA, USA

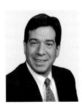

Jay S Duker MD PhD
Director, New England Eye Center
Professor and Chair of Ophthalmology
Tufts Medical Center
Tufts University School of Medicine
Cambridge, MA, USA

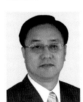

Jay Wei
Founder and CEO
Optovue, Inc
Fremont, CA, USA

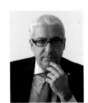

Leonardo Mastropasqua MD
Full Professor in Ophthalmology
Head
Department of Ophthalmology University
G d'Annunzio, Chieti-Pescara
Center of Excellence, National High-Tech Center
(CNAT), and Italian School of Robotic Surgery in
Ophthalmology, Italy

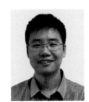

Liang Liu MD
Casey Eye Institute
Oregon Health and Science University
Portland, USA

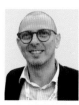
Luca Di Antonio MD PhD
Retina Fellow
Department of Ophthalmology University
G d'Annunzio
Chieti-Pescara, Italy

Maddalena Quaranta-El Maftouhi MD
Centre Rabelais
Lyon, France

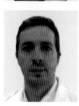
Marco Bonini Filho MD PhD
New England Eye Center
Tufts Medical Center
Tufts University School of Medicine
Boston, MA, USA

Marco Rispoli MD
Staff Ophthalmologist
Department of Ophthalmology
Ospedale Nuova Regina Margherita
Centro Italiano Macula
Rome, Italy

Maria Cristina Savastano MD PhD
Catholic University of Rome
Centro Italiano Macula
Rome, Italy

Matthew Olson CRA
Director, Ocular Imaging Service
Department of Ophthalmology
University of Mississippi Medical Center
Mississippi, USA

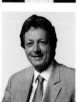
Michel Puech MD FRSC
Explore Vision, Paris
VuExplore Institute, Rueil-Malmaison
France

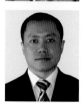
Min Wang MD PhD
Professor
Department of Ophthalmology
Eye and ENT Hospital of Fudan University
Shanghai, China

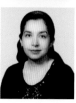
Nadia K Waheed MD MPH
Assistant Professor, Ophthalmology
Tufts University School of Medicine
Boston, MA, USA

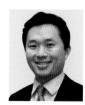
Royce Chen MD
Assistant Professor of Clinical Ophthalmology
Associate Residency Program Director
Vitreoretinal Surgery and Uveitis
Edward S Harkness Eye Institute
Columbia University Medical Center
New York, USA

Rubens Belfort Jr MD
President, Vision Institute
Head Professor
Federal University of Sao Paulo
Sao Paulo, Brazil

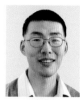
Simon S Gao PhD
Postdoctoral Fellow
Casey Eye Institute
Oregon Heath and Science University
Portland, USA

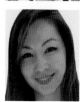
Talisa de Carlo BA
Fellow, New England Eye Center
Tufts Medical Center
Tufts University School of Medicine
Boston, MA, USA

Tony Ko
Vice-President of Research and Development
Optovue, Inc.
Fremont, CA, USA

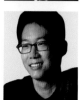
WooJhon Choi PhD
Engineer
Department of Electrical Engineering and
Research Laboratory of Electronics
Massachusetts Institute of Technology
Cambridge, MA, USA

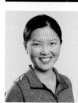
Yali Jia PhD
Research Assistant Professor
Casey Eye Institute
Oregon Health and Science University
Portland, USA

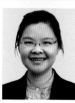
Yan Li PhD
Research Assistant Professor
Casey Eye Institute
Oregon Health and Science University
Portland, USA

Foreword

The *Clinical OCT Angiography Atlas* is a foremost guide for the understanding and interpretation of the powerful new imaging modality of OCT angiography or angio OCT. All the authors, Bruno Lumbroso, David Huang, Ching J Chen, Marco Rispoli, André Romano, Yali Jia and Nadia K Waheed have assembled and edited this landmark publication which includes contributions from internationally leading clinicians and researchers in ophthalmology and optical coherence tomography imaging.

OCT angiography is a new functional imaging modality for clinical ophthalmology and fundamental research. OCT angiography visualizes microvasculature by detecting motion contrast from blood flow. Unlike traditional fluorescein or indocyanine green angiography, it does not require injected contrast agents. Therefore, OCT angiography cannot detect vascular permeability changes which are manifested as dye leakage in traditional angiography, however, it can generate higher quality images because visualization is not impaired by diffuse hyperfluorescence. OCT angiography examinations can be performed rapidly, without patient discomfort and repeatedly; potentially on every patient visit to assess progression or treatment response.

OCT angiography uses high speed OCT structural imaging and provides three-dimensional data on microvascular structure, enabling separate *en face* visualization of retinal capillary plexuses as well as choriocapillaris, combined with coregistered *en face* and cross-sectional structural OCT. Although OCT angiography is a powerful modality, it can have imaging artifacts and provides information that is inherently more complex than structural OCT alone. Successful interpretation of OCT angiography findings requires an understanding of how OCT angiography works, the association of different ocular pathologies with their angiographic features, and integrated assessment of angiographic and structural OCT image data.

Consisting of more than 20 chapters, the *Clinical OCT Angiography Atlas* describes OCT angiography technology, methods and image interpretation. It provides a guide for interpreting OCT angiography in macular disease; covering age-related macular degeneration, diabetic retinopathy, macular telangictasia, myopia and other pathologies, as well as glaucoma and choroidal imaging. The atlas also discusses ongoing research in OCT angiography and its potential for future clinical practice. The *Clinical OCT Angiography Atlas* is an invaluable and comprehensive reference for clinicians and researchers to understand, interpret, and utilize this exciting new ophthalmic imaging modality.

James G Fujimoto PhD
Elihu Thomson Professor
Electrical Engineering and Computer Science
Massachusetts Institute of Technology
Cambridge, MA, USA

Preface

OCT angiography is a new high resolution imaging method for visualizing the retinal and choroidal circulation without the injection of any dye. By rapidly detecting intravascular flow when needed and being able to repeat the images, as often as necessary, at no risk to the patient, clinicians will come to appreciate OCT angiography as one of the most important applications of *en face* OCT imaging because of its ability to offer precise visualization of intravascular flow in the inner and outer retinal layers, as well as the inner choroid. An added advantage of this imaging strategy is that the same images acquired during OCT angiography can also be viewed as typical OCT B-scans. While it is no longer the domain of just a few privileged researchers and retina specialists, OCT angiography is now widely available to eye practitioners. As the quality of OCT angiography imaging improves and its availability becomes even more widespread, we predict that this noninvasive technology will become a new standard for imaging both the retinal and choroidal vasculature and anatomy.

The aim of this *Clinical OCT Angiography Atlas* is to show OCT users the utility of *clinical* OCT angiography imaging. The keyword is 'clinical'. We hope to develop interest in the use of OCT angiography in everyday clinical activities and help users interpret OCT angiographic images. The operating principles and the future of OCT angiography are explained by some of the original developers of the technology, and well-known authors from around the world wrote the clinical chapters. This atlas should guide the general ophthalmologists to select the best OCT angiographic views and to be able to identify the typical and atypical features of the OCT angiographic images.

The everyday use of OCT angiographic imaging in the clinics has already generated enormous interest and its importance will grow rapidly in the next few years. Our atlas is designed to appeal a wide audience with interest in a variety disorders. We hope that this atlas fulfills a huge unmet clinical need to learn more about OCT angiography.

Bruno Lumbroso
David Huang
Ching J Chen
Yali Jia
Marco Rispoli
André Romano
Nadia K Waheed

Contents

PART 1

Technology and Interpretation

Section Outline

Section 1: Methods and Techniques of OCT Angiography Examination
- Principles of Optical Coherence Tomography Angiography
- Interpretation of Optical Coherence Tomography Angiography
- Optical Coherence Tomography Angiography: Terminology
- Techniques for Using OCT Angiography for Clinical Examination
- Clinical Applications of OCT SSADA Angiography in Everyday Clinical Practice

Section 2: OCT Angiography Examination of Structure and Histology
- Retinal Normal Vascularization

Principles of Optical Coherence Tomography Angiography

David Huang, Yali Jia, Simon S Gao

INTRODUCTION

Optical coherence tomography (OCT) has become part of the standard of care in ophthalmology. It provides cross-sectional and three-dimensional (3D) imaging of the anterior segment, retina, and optic nerve head with micrometer-scale depth resolution. Structural OCT enhances the clinician's ability to detect and monitor fluid exudation associated with vascular diseases. It, however, is unable to directly detect capillary dropout or pathologic vessel growth (neovascularization) that constitutes the major vascular change associated with two leading causes of blindness, age-related macular degeneration and diabetic retinopathy. These features, among other vascular abnormalities, are assessed clinically using fluorescein or indocyanine green (ICG) angiography. To overcome conventional structural OCT's inability to provide direct blood flow information, several OCT angiography methods have been developed.

OCT ANGIOGRAPHY

Initially, Doppler OCT angiography methods were investigated for the visualization and measurement of blood flow.[1-6] Because Doppler OCT is sensitive only to motion parallel to the OCT probe beam, it is limited in its ability to image retinal and choroidal circulation, which are predominantly perpendicular to the OCT beam. An alternative approach has been speckle based OCT angiography. It has advantages over Doppler-based techniques because it uses the variation of the speckle pattern in time to detect both transverse and axial flow with similar sensitivities. Amplitude-based,[7-9] phase-based,[10] or combined amplitude + phase[11] variance methods have been described.

Split-Spectrum Amplitude: Decorrelation Angiography

We developed an amplitude-based method called split-spectrum amplitude-decorrelation angiography (SSADA). The SSADA algorithm detects motion in blood vessel lumen by measuring the variation in reflected OCT signal amplitude between consecutive cross-sectional scans. Decorrelation is a mathematical function that quantifies variation without being affected by the average signal strength, as long as the signal is strong enough to predominate over optical and electronic noise. This novelty of SSADA lies in how the OCT signal is processed to enhance flow detection and reject axial bulk motion noise. Specifically, the algorithm splits the OCT image into different spectral bands, thus increasing the number of usable image frames. Each new frame has a lower axial resolution that is less susceptible to axial eye motion caused by retrobulbar pulsation. This lower resolution also translates to a wider coherence gate over which reflected signal from a moving particle such as a blood cell can interfere with adjacent structures, thereby increasing speckle contrast. In addition, each spectral band contains a different speckle pattern and independent information on flow. When amplitude decorrelation images from multiple spectral bands are combined, the flow signal is increased. Compared to the full-spectrum amplitude method, SSADA using four-fold spectral splits improved the signal-to-noise ratio (SNR) by a factor of two, which is equivalent to reducing the scan time by a factor of four.[12] More recent SSADA implementations use even more than a four-fold split to further enhance the SNR of flow detection. As shown by an example from *en face* angiograms of the macular retinal circulation collected using a commercial 70 kHz 840 nm spectral OCT (Figs 1.1A to H), SSADA provides a clean and continuous microvascular network and less noise just inside the foveal avascular zone (FAZ).

Since OCT angiography generates 3D data, segmentation and *en face* presentation of the flow information can aid in reducing data complexity and serve to reproduce the more traditional view of dye-based angiography. As seen in Figure 1.1, the retinal angiogram (Figs 1.1B to D) represents the decorrelation or flow information between the internal limiting membrane and the outer plexiform layer. Segmentation performed on the cross-

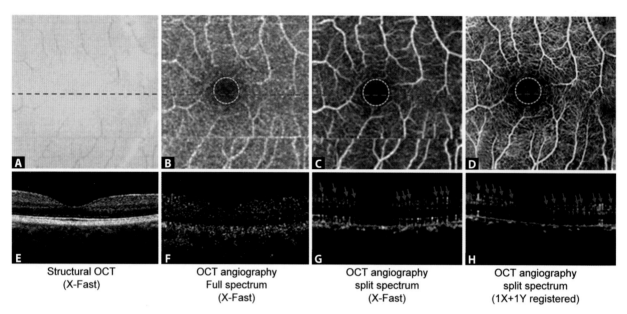

| Structural OCT (X-Fast) | OCT angiography Full spectrum (X-Fast) | OCT angiography split spectrum (X-Fast) | OCT angiography split spectrum (1X+1Y registered) |

Figs 1.1A to H: Comparison of structural OCT (A, E) and amplitude-decorrelation angiograms of the macula (3 × 3 mm area) using full spectrum (B, F), split-spectrum (C, G), and split-spectrum averaged angiograms from one X-fast and one F-fast scans after 3D registration (D, H). *En face* maximum decorrelation projections of retinal circulation showed less noise inside the foveal avascular zone (FAZ, within green dotted circles) and more continuous perifoveal vascular networks using the SSADA algorithm (C) compared to standard full-spectrum algorithm (B). The cross-sectional angiograms (scanned across the red dashed line in B and C) showed more clearly delineated retinal vessels (red arrows in G) and less noise using the SSADA algorithm (G) compared to the standard (F). There are saccadic motion artifacts that appear as artifactual horizontal lines in (B, C). This and other motion artifacts are removed using the 3D registration algorithm that registers a horizontal-priority (X-fast) and a vertical-priority (Y-fast) raster scans to remove motion error. The algorithm then merges the X-fast and Y-fast scans to produce a merged 3D OCT angiogram that shows a continuous artifact-free microvascular network in (D). The registration and averaging of two orthogonal scans also removed motion blur and further improved SNR, allowing the visualization of a greater number of distinct small retinal vessels (microvascular network in D, red arrows in H).

sectional, structural OCT images (Fig. 1.1E) can directly be applied to the OCT angiography images (Figs 1.1F and G). The *en face* angiograms were generated by projecting the maximum decorrelation or flow value for each transverse position within the segmented depth range, representing the fastest flowing vessel lumen in the segmented tissue layers. In healthy eyes, the retinal angiogram shows a vascular network around the FAZ. The layers of the retina and choroid can be more finely separated to provide additional information to define diagnostic parameters of vascular defects. This will be discussed in Chapter 2.

Relationship Between Decorrelation and Velocity

To determine how the decorrelation or flow signal produced by the SSADA algorithm relates to flow velocity, phantom experiments were performed.[13] The study showed that SSADA is sensitive to both axial and transverse flow, with a slightly higher sensitivity for the axial component. For clinical retinal imaging where the OCT beam is approximately perpendicular to the vasculature, the SSADA signal can be considered to be independent of the small variation in beam incidence angle for all practical purposes. In addition, it was found that decorrelation was linearly related to velocity over a limited range. A higher decorrelation value thus implies higher velocity flow. This range is dependent on the time scale of the SSADA measurement. With a 70 kHz spectral OCT system and 200+ A-scans per cross-sectional B-scan, SSADA should be sensitive to even the slowest flow at the capillary

level, where flow speeds have been estimated at between 0.4 to 3 mm/s.[14,15] In larger vessels with higher velocities, the SSADA signal reaches a maximum value (saturates).

Comparison to Fluorescein and Indocyanine Green Angiography

Compared to fluorescein or ICG angiography, the gold standards of retinal vascular imaging, OCT angiography has a number of advantages and differences. SSADA can be acquired in a few seconds and does not require intravenous injection, whereas fluorescein or ICG angiography requires multiple image frames taken over several minutes and can cause nausea, vomiting, and, albeit rarely, anaphylaxis.[16] The fast and noninvasive nature of OCT angiography also means that follow-up scans can be conducted more frequently.

Dye leakage in fluorescein angiography is the hallmark of important vascular abnormalities such as neovascularization and microaneurysms. OCT angiography does not employ a dye and cannot evaluate leakage. OCT angiography detects vascular abnormalities by other methods based on depth and vascular pattern. Choroidal neovascularization is characterized by distinct vascular patterns present above the retinal pigment epithelium (Type II) or between the Bruch's membrane and the retinal pigment epithelium (Type I). Because dye leakage and staining do not occur in OCT angiography, the boundaries, and therefore areas, of capillary dropout and neovascularization can be more precisely measured. The visualization of intraretinal and subretinal fluid accumulation on structural OCT may provide information analogous to fluid leakage. Thus, although the lack of dye leakage is a limitation of OCT angiography, other ways of detecting vascular abnormality more than make up for this deficit. Furthermore, conventional angiography is two-dimensional, which makes it difficult to distinguish vascular abnormalities within different layers. The 3D nature of OCT angiography allows for separate evaluation of abnormalities in the retinal and choroidal circulations.

Limitations of Optical Coherence Tomography Angiography

OCT angiography has several limitations. First, shadowgraphic flow projection artifact makes the interpretation of *en face* angiograms of deeper vascular beds more difficult. These artifacts are a result of fluctuating shadows cast by flowing blood in a superficial vascular layer that cause variation of the OCT signal in deeper, highly reflective layers. The flow projection artifact from the retinal circulation can be seen clearly on the bright retinal pigment epithelium (RPE). This artifact can be removed by software processing. The projection from the retinal circulation is relatively sparse and can be removed from deeper layers fairly effectively. However, the choriocapillaris is nearly confluent, and its projection and shadow effects are difficult to remove from deeper choroidal layers. A second limitation is the fading of OCT and flow signal in large vessels due to the interferometric fringe washout effect associated with very fast blood flow, especially the axial flow component.[17] This means that central retinal vessels in the disc and large vessels in the deep choroid cannot be visualized using SSADA. Third, the scan area of OCT angiography is relatively small (3×3 to 6×6 mm). Larger-area angiograms of high quality can be achieved, but require higher speed OCT systems that are not yet commercially available.[18]

Lastly, because OCT angiography best resolves pathology when viewed as *en face* angiograms of anatomic layers, practical clinical applications require accurate segmentation software. Post-processing software is also needed to reduce motion and projection artifacts. The need for these sophisticated algorithms means OCT angiography still has much room to improve in the foreseeable future.

COMPARING SWEPT-SOURCE AND SPECTRAL OPTICAL COHERENCE TOMOGRAPHY

The SSADA algorithm was initially implemented on a custom-built 100 kHz 1050 nm wavelength swept-source OCT system. To generate high quality angiograms (Fig. 1.2A), 8 consecutive cross-sectional scans at each position were necessary. A scan pattern of 200 cross-sectional scan positions each with 200 axial scans was used. The overall angiographic scan pattern had 200 × 200 transverse points. 200 × 200 × 8 axial scans were acquired in 3.5 seconds.

The commercial implementation of SSADA uses a 70 kHz 840 nm wavelength spectral OCT system (RTVue XR Avanti, Optovue, Inc., Fremont, CA). Although the systems acquire fewer axial scans per second, high quality angiograms with more transverse points (304 × 304, Fig. 1.2B) are produced in less time (2.9 seconds). The higher performance is due to the lower decorrelation noise on the spectral OCT system, which only requires 2 consecutive cross-sectional scans at one position to compute a reliable decorrelation image. The higher transverse scan density, along with a higher transverse resolution associated with the shorter wavelength, means that the Avanti produces retinal angiograms with higher definition and higher resolution than the swept-source OCT prototype we originally used (Figs 1.2 C and D).

Swept-source OCT   **Spectral OCT**

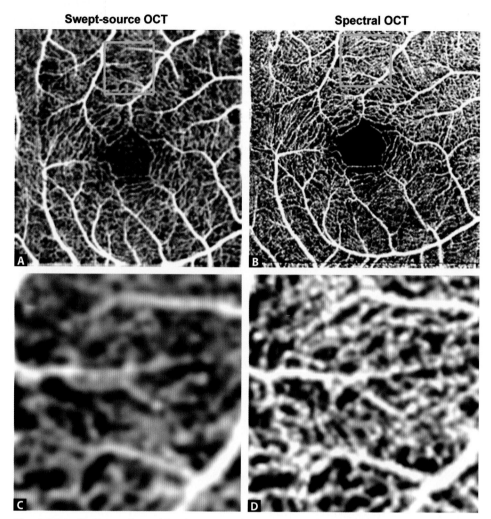

Figs 1.2A to D: Comparison of 3 × 3 mm macular angiograms from a 100 kHz swept-source OCT system (A) and 70 kHz spectral OCT system (B). Zoomed-in views shows improve capillary detail from the spectral OCT system (D) as compared to the swept-source OCT system (C).

REFERENCES

1. Wang RK, et al. Three dimensional optical angiography. Opt Express. 2007;15:4083-97.

2. Grulkowski I, et al. Scanning protocols dedicated to smart velocity ranging in Spectral OCT. Opt Express. 2009;17:23736-54.

3. Yu L, Chen Z. Doppler variance imaging for three-dimensional retina and choroid angiography. J Biomed Opt. 2010;15:016029.

4. Makita S, Jaillon F, Yamanari M, Miura M, Yasuno Y. Comprehensive in vivo micro-vascular imaging of the human eye by dual-beam-scan Doppler optical coherence angiography. Optics Express. 2011;19:1271-83.

5. Zotter S, et al. Visualization of microvasculature by dual-beam phase-resolved Doppler optical coherence tomography. Optics Express. 2011; 19:1217-27.

6. Braaf B, Vermeer KA, Vienola KV, de Boer JF. Angiography of the retina and the choroid with phase-resolved OCT using interval-optimized backstitched B-scans. Optics Express. 2012;20:20516-34.

7. Mariampillai A, et al. Speckle variance detection of microvasculature using swept-source optical coherence tomography. Opt Lett. 2008;33: 1530-2.

8. Motaghiannezam R, Fraser S. Logarithmic intensity and speckle-based motion contrast methods for human retinal vasculature visualization using swept source optical coherence tomography. Biomed. Opt Express. 2012;3:503-21.

9. Enfield J, Jonathan E, Leahy M. In vivo imaging of the microcirculation of the volar forearm using correlation mapping optical coherence tomography (cmOCT). Biomed. Opt Express. 2011;2:1184-93.

10. Fingler J, Zawadzki RJ, Werner JS, Schwartz D, Fraser SE. Volumetric microvascular imaging of human retina using optical coherence tomography with a novel motion contrast technique. Opt Express. 2009; 17:22190-200.

11. Liu G, Lin AJ, Tromberg BJ, Chen Z. A comparison of Doppler optical coherence tomography methods. Biomed. Opt Express. 2012;3:2669-80.

12. Jia Y, et al. Split-spectrum amplitude-decorrelation angiography with optical coherence tomography. Opt Express. 2012;20:4710-25.

13. Tokayer J, Jia Y, Dhalla AH, Huang D. Blood flow velocity quantification using split-spectrum amplitude-decorrelation angiography with

optical coherence tomography. Biomed Opt Express. 2013;4:1909-24, doi:10.1364/BOE.4.001909 193860 [pii].

14. Riva CE, Petrig B. Blue field entoptic phenomenon and blood velocity in the retinal capillaries. J Opt Soc Am. 1980;70:1234-8.

15. Tam J, Tiruveedhula P, Roorda A. Characterization of single-file flow through human retinal parafoveal capillaries using an adaptive optics scanning laser ophthalmoscope. Biomed Opt Express. 2011;2:781-93, doi:10.1364/BOE.2.000781.

16. Lopez-Saez M, et al. Fluorescein-induced allergic reaction. Annals of Allergy, Asthma and Immunology. 1998;81:428-30 .

17. Hendargo HC, McNabb RP, Dhalla AH, Shepherd N, Izatt JA. Doppler velocity detection limitations in spectrometer-based versus swept-source optical coherence tomography. Biomedical Optics Express. 2011;2:2175-88.

18. Blatter C, et al. Ultrahigh-speed non-invasive widefield angiography. BIOMEDO. 2012;17:0705051-3.

Interpretation of Optical Coherence Tomography Angiography

David Huang, Yali Jia, Simon S Gao

This chapter refers to optical coherence tomography (OCT) angiography performed using the split-spectrum amplitude decorrelation angiography (SSADA) algorithm on either a swept-source OCT prototype or a commercial spectral OCT system (RTVue-XR Avanti, Optovue, Inc., Fremont, CA). But generally the principles are also applicable to other types of OCT angiography.

ANATOMIC REFERENCE PLANES AND ANGIOGRAPHIC SLABS

Optical coherence tomography (OCT) angiography produces three-dimensional (3D) flow data that requires segmentation into different layers to optimally evaluate abnormalities. Computer segmentation of OCT images provides the reference planes or surface. Appropriate tissue layers or "slabs" are then defined relative to these reference planes. The useful reference planes include the inner limiting membrane (ILM), outer boundary of the inner plexiform layer (IPL), outer boundary of the outer plexiform layer (OPL), and Bruch's membrane (BM). Automated algorithms perform well in identifying these reference planes in scans of healthy eyes. However, in cases where the retina is deformed, manual correction of the reference planes or adjustment of slab boundaries may be required.

Cross-sectional OCT angiograms combine color-coded decorrelation or flow information superimposed on gray-scale reflectance signal (Fig. 2.1A). Using this technique, both blood flow and retinal structural information are presented together. This is useful to provide detailed information on the depth of abnormalities such as retinal or choroidal neovascularization.

En face presentation of OCT angiography helps clinicians recognize vascular patterns associated with various vascular abnormalities. *En face* angiograms are generated by summarizing the flow information within the depth range encompassed by relevant anatomic layers (slab), typically by taking the maximum or average decorrelation (representing flow) value. This projection process compresses the three-dimensional (3D) angiogram into

several 2D images that can be more easily interpreted. Using the segmentation of the ILM, outer boundary of the IPL, outer boundary of the OPL, retinal pigment epithelium (RPE), and BM, the following slabs can be visualized:

- **Vitreous**—normally avascular (above the ILM)
- **Superficial retinal plexus**—superficial portion of the inner retina (ILM to outer boundary of the IPL)
- **Deep retinal plexus**—deep portion of the inner retina (outer boundary of the IPL to outer boundary of the OPL)
- **Inner retina**—the combination of superficial and deep retinal plexi (ILM to outer boundary of the OPL)
- **Outer retina**—normally avascular (outer boundary of the OPL to RPE)
- **Choriocapillaris**—normally near confluent (BM to 10 to 20 μm below)
- **Deeper choroid**—larger choroidal vessels (more than 20 μm below BM)
- **Choroid**—the combination of choriocapillaris and deeper choroid
- **Custom**—user defined slab that best highlights the vascular pathology.

In a healthy eye, an *en face* OCT angiogram above the ILM shows the normal, avascular vitreous (Fig. 2.1B). The inner retina shows larger vessels in the superficial plexus (Fig. 2.1C) and fine capillary network in the deep plexus (Fig. 2.1D) with no flow in the foveal avascular zone (FAZ). The outer retina should be avascular, but flow projection artifacts from the inner retina can be seen (Fig. 2.1E). The flow projection artifact occurs because flow blood in the retinal vessels cast flickering shadows that cause OCT signal fluctuation in the layers below that is recognized as flow by the OCT angiography algorithm. Amplitude/magnitude/intensity-based, phase-based and complex amplitude-based OCT angiography are all susceptible to similar flow projection artifacts. This shadowgraphic fluctuation is most noticeable in highly reflective layers such as the retinal pigment epithelium (RPE) and forms a pattern that replicates the retinal circulation

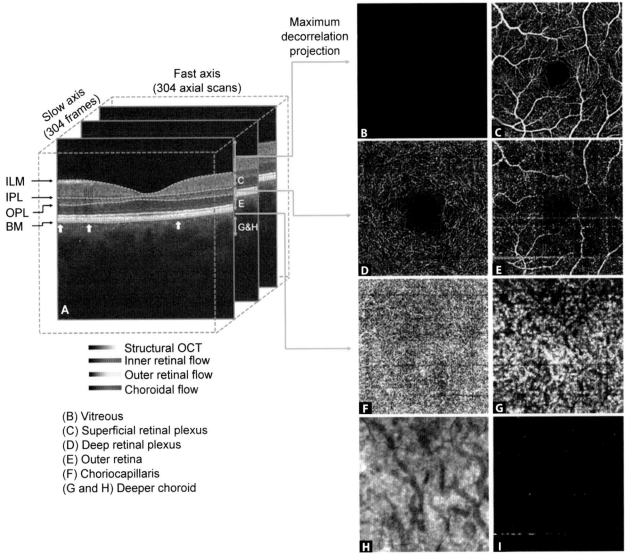

Fig. 2.1: Segmentation and processing of an OCT angiogram of a normal macula. (A) The 3D OCT angiogram comprises 304 frames of averaged decorrelation cross-sections stretched along the slow scan axis. Each frame is computed using the SSADA algorithm. The angiogram spans 3 mm in all 3 dimensions. The cross-sectional angiogram shows that flow in the inner retinal vessels (purple) are projected onto bright photoreceptor and retinal pigment epithelium (RPE) layers (indicated by white arrows). Image processing software separates the vitreous, inner retinal layers, outer retinal layer, and choroidal layers along the inner limiting membrane (ILM), outer boundary of the inner plexiform layer (IPL), outer boundary of the outer plexiform layer (OPL), and Bruch's membrane (BM) (dotted green lines). Six segmented flow volumes are separately projected. The projection algorithm finds the maximum decorrelation value for each transverse position within the segmented depth range, representing the fastest flowing vessel lumen in the segmented tissue layers. (B) The vitreous angiogram shows the absence of vascular flow. (C) The superficial inner retinal angiogram shows normal retinal circulation with a small FAZ of approximately 0.6 mm in diameter. (D) The deep inner retina angiogram shows the deep retinal plexus which is a network of fine vessels. (E) The outer retina slab shows flow projection artifacts cast by flowing blood in the inner retinal vessels onto the RPE. (F) The choriocapillaris angiogram. (G) The deeper choroid angiogram. (H) The deeper choroid *en face* structural OCT. (I) The outer retinal angiogram after removal of the projection artifact using a post-processing algorithm.

(Fig. 2.1E). The flow projection artifact can be suppressed by post-processing software (Fig. 2.1I). The choriocapillaris shows nearly confluent flow (Fig. 2.1F). Although artifactual projection of retinal vessels in the choriocapillaris is present, it is not very noticeable because the artifact is diffused by the overlying RPE and weaker than the predominant choriocapillaris circulation. Lobular structures of the choriocapillaris are difficult to recognize because it is very dense within the macula and beyond the limited transverse spatial resolution. The coarser lobules outside the macula would be recognizable. The deeper choroid angiogram shows larger vessels but is more difficult to interpret due to flow projection, shadowing, and fringe-washout artifacts. Fringe washout occurs because high flow velocity (especially the axial component) mixes the phase of the interferometric signal within the integration time of the camera or photodetector in the OCT system.[1] Together with shadowing, fringe washout can reduce OCT signal intensity below that needed for SSADA processing. Therefore, part of or entire large choroidal vessels can appear dark on both *en face* OCT angiography (Fig. 2.1G) and structural OCT (Fig. 2.1H).

ANGIOVUE DEFAULT SEGMENTATION AND DISPLAY

AngioVue™ (Optovue, Inc., Fremont, CA) is currently the only OCT angiography software available on a commercially available high-speed (70 kHz axial scan repetition rate) OCT system (RTVue-XR Avanti). It uses the SSADA algorithm to detect flow, and an orthogonal registration algorithm called "Motion Correction Technology" (MCT) to remove motion artifacts. AngioVue provides a default angiographic display scheme that defines *en face* angiographic slabs relative to a simplified set of reference planes that can be reliably segmented by current software. These include the ILM, outer boundary of IPL, and the "RPE Reference," which is the best-fit surface under the retinal pigment epithelium and approximates the BM position. For the convenience of AngioVue users, the 4 default *en face* display slab definitions are provided here:

- **Superficial retinal capillary plexus**—3 μm below the ILM to 15 μm below IPL
- **Deep retinal capillary plexus**—15 to 70 μm below the IPL
- **Outer retina**—70 μm below the IPL to 30 μm below the RPE Reference
- **Choroid capillary**—30 μm to 60 μm below the RPE reference.

These definitions are optimized for the detection of common pathologies using the automated segmentation algorithm within the AngioVue software. Therefore, they are at slight variance from the idealized layer boundaries we outlined in the last section. The automatically segmented reference planes could be manually corrected, and the slab border offset could be adjusted relative to the reference planes. With these flexibilities, the user could shift the slabs to highlight any pathology. The AngioVue outer retinal slab allows for suppression of flow projection artifact from the overlying retinal blood vessel onto the RPE. This can be turned on or off with a "Remove Artifacts" check box. Artifact suppression is useful for the clean visualization of choroidal neovascularization (CNV) and is explained in more detail below.

RECOGNIZING FLOW PROJECTION ARTIFACT AND NONVASCULAR FLOW SIGNAL

Shadowgraphic flow projection artifacts result from fluctuating shadows cast by flowing blood in the large inner retinal vessels that cause variation of the OCT signal in deeper layers. Similarly, CNV component above BM could project onto choroidal layers below. This signal variation would be detected as a decorrelation and could not be differentiated from true flow-based on signal characteristics alone. The clinician can recognize the flow projection artifact by noting that it forms a vertical streak in the cross-sectional OCT angiogram (Fig. 2.1A), and that the vascular pattern of a more superficial layer is replicated on a deeper layer (Fig. 2.1E compared to 2.1C). It is particularly important not to be fooled by this artifact in the detection of CNV. The RPE is the dominant screen on which the retinal blood flow is projected. This produces a prominent flow projection artifact in the outer retinal slab that is reduced using a projection artifact suppression algorithm in the AngioVue software (Fig. 2.2). The algorithm still leaves residual patchy flow signal that are non-vascular in origin. This non-vascular flow signal is again most noticeable in highly scattering tissue (e.g. RPE). This artifact does not have the distinct patterns presented by CNV, which are described in the last section of this chapter. CNV is ruled out in this dry age-related macular degeneration (AMD) example by the absence of any distinct CNV vascular pattern in artifact-suppressed outer retina slab as well as the choriocapillaris slab.

QUANTIFICATION: FLOW INDEX AND VESSEL DENSITY

SSADA allows for the quantification of blood flow within the regions of interest. The flow index and vessel density can be determined from the *en face* maximum projection angiogram. The flow index is calculated as the average decorrelation value

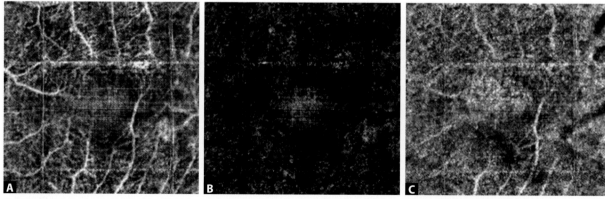

Figs 2.2A to C: Angiovue OCT aniography of an eye with dry age-related macular degeneration. (A) *En face* OCT angiogram of the outer retina shows dense flow projection from the retinal vasculature above. (B) *En face* OCT angiogram of the outer retina after application of the projection artifact removal algorithm shows residual patches of nonvascular flow signal. They can be recognized as artifact because they do not have any distinct vascular pattern. (C) En face OCT angiogram of the choriocapillaris does not show any CNV pattern.

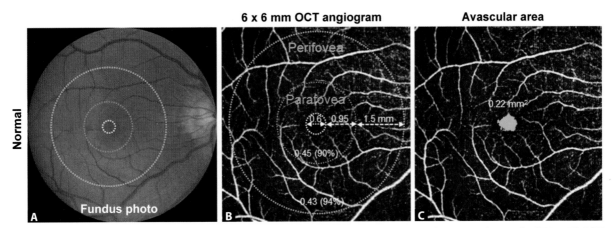

Figs 2.3A to C: Quantification of inner retinal blood flows in a normal eye using OCT angiography acquired using the RTVue-XR OCT system. White dashed circle: Normal foveal avascular zone (FAZ, 0.6 mm diameter white dashed circle). Area between white and blue dashed circles: parafoveal zone. Area between blue and green dashed circles: Perifoveal zone. (A) Fundus photo. (B) *En face* 6 × 6 mm OCT angiogram of the inner retina. Parafoveal and perifoveal retinal flow indexes (vessel densities) were calculated using custom software. (C) An avascular area (blue) was identified in the normal FAZ with area of 0.22 mm² using a custom software developed by the authors.

(which is correlated with flow velocity) in the selected region. The vessel density is calculated as the percentage area occupied by vessels and microvasculature in the selected region.

Typical Regions of Interest

For scans of the macula, flow index and vessel density can be routinely determined for the parafovea and/or perifovea. The parafovea is defined to be an annular region with an inner diameter of 0.6 mm and outer diameter of 2.5 mm centered on the FAZ (Fig. 2.3). The perifovea is defined to be the annular region extending from the edge of the parafovea to an outer diameter of 5.5 mm. These zones are illustrated on a 6 × 6 mm macular retinal angiogram of a normal eye in Figure 2.3B.

For scans of the optic nerve head, flow index and vessel density can be routinely determined for the peripapillary retina. The peripapillary is defined as an elliptical annulus extending outward from the optic disc boundary.

INTERPRETATION OF PATHOLOGICAL OPTICAL COHERENCE TOMOGRAPHY ANGIOGRAPHY

On OCT angiography, pathology is identified by the absence or reduction of flow in normally vascular layers or abnormal vascular patterns in normally avascular layers.

Detection of Capillary Dropout and Measurement of Nonperfusion Area

OCT angiography can visualize areas of capillary dropout. In a normal eye (Fig. 2.3), the retinal capillary network is dense with the exception of the FAZ, where capillaries are normally absent. In an eye with proliferative diabetic retinopathy (Fig. 2.4), areas of nonperfusion could be identified outside of the FAZ using custom software.

Detection of Retinal Neovascularization

The development of retinal neovascularization (RNV) signifies progression to the proliferative case of diabetic retinopathy. The recognition of RNV is important as it may guide the treatment decision regarding panretinal photocoagulation which has been shown to reduce the risk of vision loss due to RNV.[2] OCT angiography can be used to distinguish between intraretinal microvascular abnormalities, which occupy the same plane as the retinal blood vessels, and early RNV, which develops anterior to the ILM (Fig. 2.4). The extent and activity of RNV can also be quantified on OCT angiography by flow index and vessel area. The commercial AngioVue software does not have a default vitreous slab currently, but the user could obtain such a view by manually shifting the superficial retinal plexus slab upward.

Detection of Choroidal Neovascularization

Choroidal neovascularization (CNV), the primary pathologic feature of neovascular AMD, consists of abnormal blood vessels growth from the choriocapillaris. The CNV penetrate through BM into the subretinal pigment epithelium (RPE) space and subretinal space. Subsequent exudation and hemorrhage damage retinal tissues, resulting in vision loss.[3] Detection and classification of CNV as Type I or II relies on proper segmentation. Examples using Optovue's AngioVue software are shown.

In an example of Type I CNV (Fig. 2.5), absence of the CNV in the outer retinal slab above the RPE and presence of the CNV in the slab below the RPE establishes it as Type I. Because Type I CNV is below the RPE, it projects very well into the choroidal slab. Thus the choroidal slab is an excellent view for Type I CNV detection. However, one must keep in mind that the CNV network visualized in the *en face* OCT angiogram of the choroidal slab includes a projected component that is above the BM, as well as the true choroidal component below the BM.

In an example of Type II CNV (Fig. 2.6), the abnormal vessels are well visualized in the default AngioVue outer retinal slab. To

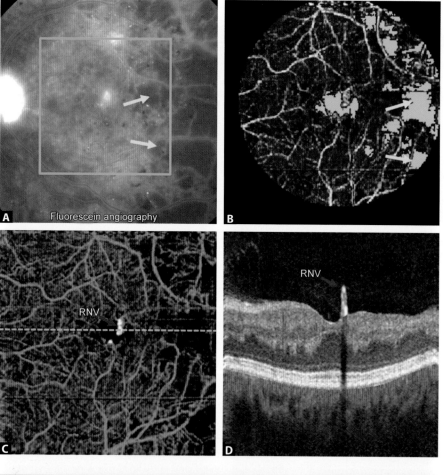

Figs 2.4A to D: Proliferative diabetic retinopathy imaged using RTVue-XR AngioVue and processed with custom software. (A) Late frame fluorescein angiogram showing numerous microaneurysms, hyperfluorescence at the fovea, and regions of hypofluoresence temporal to the fovea (yellow arrows). The green square outlines the 6 × 6 mm area shown on the OCT angiogram. (B) Avascular areas (blue) were identified on the inner retinal *en face* OCT angiogram using custom software. (C) Composite *en face* OCT angiogram showing flow signal of retinal neovascularization (RNV, yellow) above the inner limit membrane (ILM) on a background of retinal vessels (purple). (D) Cross-sectional OCT angiogram RNV (yellow) above the ILM. Inner retinal flow is in purple; choroidal flow is in red.

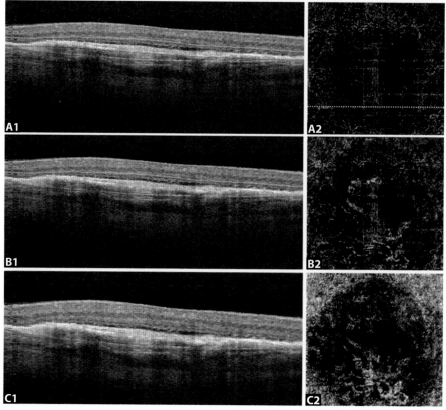

Figs 2.5A to C: (A1) Cross-sectional structural OCT image showing the upper (green) and lower (red) boundaries of the outer retinal slab as defined by the default AngioVue software segmentation. It includes the RPE and above. (A2) *En face* angiogram of the outer retina as defined by the segmentation in (A1) showing no CNV. The blue dotted line shows the location of (A1). (B1) The same structural image with the lower boundary of the slab moved 100 µm lower to the level of the BM; (B2) The resulting angiogram reveals the presence of Type I CNV. The AngioVue software was set to remove flow projection artifacts from these angiograms of the outer retinal slab. (C1) Cross-sectional structural OCT showing the borders of the choroidal slab at 30 and 60 µm below a manually corrected RPE Reference. (C2) *En face* OCT angiogram of the choroidal slab shows the CNV well.

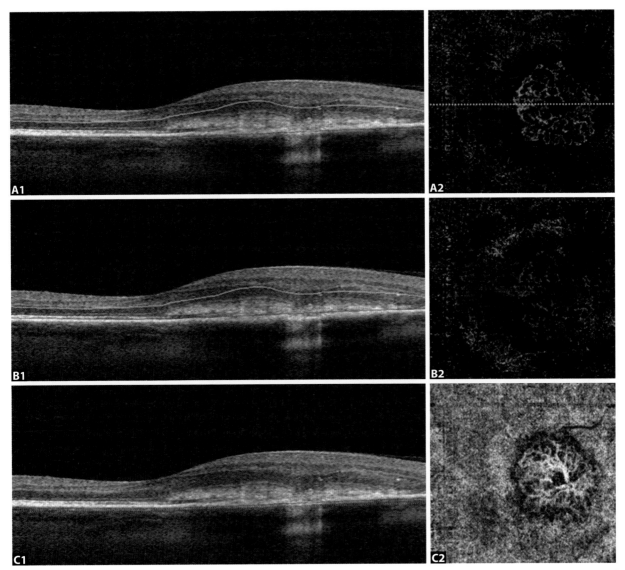

Figs 2.6A to C: (A1) Cross-sectional structural OCT image showing the upper (green) and lower (red) boundaries of the outer retina slab as defined by the default AngioVue software segmentation. (A2) *En face* angiogram of the outer retinal slab reveals CNV. The blue dotted line shows the location of (A1). (B1) The same structural image with the lower boundary of the outer retinal slab adjusted 47 μm upward to a level just above the RPE. (B2) The resulting angiogram shows that the CNV exists above the RPE. The AngioVue software was set to remove flow projection artifacts from these angiograms of the outer retinal slab. (C1) Cross-sectional structural OCT showing the borders of the choroidal slab at 30 and 60 μm below RPE Reference. (C2) *En face* OCT angiogram of the choroidal slab clearly shows the CNV.

determine whether the CNV has a component above the RPE, it is necessary to move the lower boundary of the slab above the RPE to see if the CNV can still be visualized. In this case, much of the CNV vessel pattern remains, thus classifying this case as Type II CNV. Note that the CNV pattern appears brighter in the choroidal slab because it was not filtered by the artifact removal algorithm. But the CNV patterns appears the same both in the inner retinal slab and the choroidal slab, indicating that the CNV pattern in the choroid mostly represents projection from CNV above the BM, and not a large CNV component below the BM. Also note a dark shroud surrounding the CNV in the choroidal slab in both examples of type I (Fig. 2.5) and type II (Fig. 2.6) CNV. This is a common appearance that might indicate choroid defect in the region of the CNV.

Because retinal flow projection onto the outer retina slab can make it difficult to identify CNV, a color composite scheme can be used to aid in visualization (Fig. 2.7).[4] In this example, a composite *en face* angiogram (Fig. 2.7H) shows the superficial retinal circulation (Fig. 2.7D) in purple and the outer retinal flow (Fig. 2.7E) in yellow. Areas of subretinal fluid are also shown in blue. Displaying the volumetric flow information as a composite image is advantageous as the retinal circulation in purple would mask the flow projection seen in the outer retina. In addition, it allows for identification of the CNV relative to landmarks in the superficial retinal vasculature.

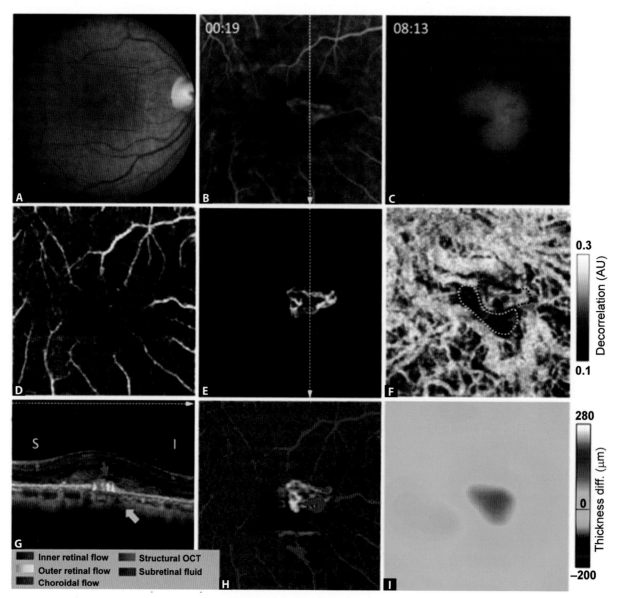

Figs 2.7A to I: AMD patient with type I choroidal neovascularization (CNV). (A) Color fundus photograph showing subretinal hemorrhage. Red square outlines the area shown on angiograms below; (B) Early-phase fluorescein angiography (FA); (C) Late-phase FA; (D) *En face* optical coherence tomography (OCT) angiogram of the inner retina. (E) *En face* angiogram of the outer retina showing the CNV. The yellow dashed lines indicate the position of OCT cross-section shown in (G). Yellow arrows indicate the superior to inferior direction; (F) *En face* angiogram of the choroid showing patchy flow directly under the CNV (blue dotted outline) and an adjacent area of reduced flow (green dotted outline). (G) Cross-sectional color OCT angiogram showing the CNV (yellow) was predominantly under the retinal pigment epithelial (RPE). The blue arrow shows the location of the subretinal fluid. The green arrow corresponds to the green dashed outline in (F) showing a focal region of reduced choroidal flow adjacent to the CNV. I = inferior; S = superior; (H) Composite *en face* OCT angiograms showing most subretinal fluid (dark blue) inferior to the CNV; (I) Retinal thickness deviation map showing retinal thickening over the CNV.
Source: From reference 4.

REFERENCES

1. Hendargo HC, McNabb RP, Dhalla AH, Shepherd N, Izatt JA. Doppler velocity detection limitations in spectrometer-based versus swept-source optical coherence tomography. Biomedical Optics Express. 2011;2: 2175-88.

2. Group DRSR. Photocoagulation treatment of proliferative diabetic retinopathy: Clinical application of diabetic retinopathy study (DRS) findings, DRS report number 8. Ophthalmology. 1981;88:583-600.

3. Ambati J, Ambati BK, Yoo SH, Lanchulev S, Adamis AP. Age-related macular degeneration: Etiology, pathogenesis, and therapeutic strategies. Survey of Ophthalmology. 2003;48:257-293, doi:10.1016/s0039-6257(03)00030-4.

4. Jia Y, et al. Quantitative optical coherence tomography angiography of choroidal neovascularization in age-related macular degeneration. Ophthalmology. 2014;121:1435-44. doi:10.1016/j.ophtha.2014.01.034 S0161-6420(14)00104-3 [pii].

Optical Coherence Tomography Angiography: Terminology

David Huang, Yali Jia, Simon S Gao

STRUCTURAL OPTICAL COHERENCE TOMOGRAPHY

This is the conventional use of optical coherence tomography (OCT) systems where the OCT signal intensity representing tissue reflectance is displayed in gray-scale or pseudocolor scale to provide structural information with micron resolution.

Reflectance

Reflectance is a property of the tissue structure that affects the amount of light backscattered or reflected by the tissue sample. It is primarily caused by variation of refractive index within tissue microstructure. Light attenuation due to tissue scattering and absorption also affect the amount of light detected by OCT.

Signal Intensity or Amplitude

Signal intensity and amplitude both refer to the amount of light detected by the OCT system. Intensity is related to the power reflected from the sample and optical field amplitude or magnitude is related to the square root of the intensity. For example, the retinal pigment epithelium (RPE) is more reflective than surrounding tissues. Thus, it produces a strong OCT signal and appears brighter on structural OCT images.

OPTICAL COHERENCE TOMOGRAPHY ANGIOGRAPHY

OCT angiography refers to a variety of techniques designed to image vascular patterns in tissue. Originally an offshoot of Doppler OCT that detects only axial flow, most recent implementations assess variations in speckle amplitude and/or phase in order to detect both transverse and axial flow.

Amplitude/Magnitude/Intensity Variance

These refer to methods which detect motion or flow by looking for change in the OCT signal over time as measured by the variance or decorrelation of signal amplitude (*aka* magnitude), intensity, or their log transforms.

Phase Variance

Phase variance uses changes in the phase of the OCT signal as the means of detecting flow.

Split-spectrum Amplitude-decorrelation Angiography

Split-spectrum amplitude-decorrelation angiography (SSADA) is an efficient algorithm which improves the signal-to-noise ratio of flow detection by maximizing the extraction of flow information from speckle variation. This is achieved by splitting the OCT spectrum, which increases the number of usable image frames and reduces noise from axial bulk motion.[1]

Amplitude Decorrelation or Flow Signal

Decorrelation is a way to quantify variations in the OCT signal amplitude without being affected by the average signal strength. The decorrelation value ranges from 0 (no variation) to 1 (maximum variation). A higher decorrelation value implies higher flow velocity, up to a limit.[2] The slowest flow that can be detected by SSADA is the *sensitivity limit*, while the *saturation limit* is the fastest flow beyond which the decorrelation value cannot increase further. The linear range lies between the sensitivity and saturation limits. The decorrelation value is also referred to as the flow signal in OCT angiography.

AngioVue

AngioVue™ is the software developed by Optovue, Inc. to perform OCT angiography on the RTVue-XR Avanti spectral OCT system. It combines the SSADA algorithm to detect flow and orthogonal 3D image registration technology to reduce motion error.

ANALYSIS OF OPTICAL COHERENCE TOMOGRAPHY ANGIOGRAPHY

Segmentation

OCT angiography produces volumetric flow information. To allow for rapid identification and interpretation of pathological vascular features, segmentation of key anatomic layers is required. Segmentation is typically performed on the structural OCT images. Key reference surfaces at the inner limiting membrane (ILM), outer boundary of the inner plexiform layer (IPL), outer boundary of the outer plexiform layer (OPL), retinal pigment epithelium (RPE), and Bruch's membrane (BM) are used to define important retinal and choroidal layers or "slabs".

Because automated algorithms will not always produce accurate segmentation, manual correction may be required. Instead of tracing the structures, which may be time consuming, offsetting the automated segmentation to better capture the region of interest is a viable alternative. In this case, positive offset values move the segmentation posteriorly, while negative offset values move anteriorly.

En Face Projection

En face projection produces two-dimensional (2D) views of segmented tissue layers. *En face* structural OCT images are typically generated by projecting the average reflectance signal intensity over depth onto a 2D canvas. *En face* angiograms are generated by projecting the maximum or average decorrelation value (flow signal) onto a 2D canvas.

Slabs and Slices

These refer to the tissue volume used for *en face* projection. Slabs refer to thick tissue sections such as the inner retina or outer retina, whereas slices refer to thin sections of a few microns used to examine fine details.

Nonvascular Flow Signal

In OCT angiography, background bulk tissue motion can generally be subtracted because it is associated with a uniform decorrelation or variance value over most voxels with measurable OCT signal. However, the decorrelation signal in some very highly backscattering structures can still rise above the background in some instances. These include the RPE, hard exudates, regions of pigment accumulation, thrombosed aneurysms, and retinal hemorrhages. Possibly, the presence of a high concentration of backscattering particles can enhance decorrelation caused by tissue movement or scanner displacement between repeated scans.

Flow Projection Artifact

Shadowgraphic flow projection artifacts are the result of fluctuating shadows cast by flowing blood in a superficial vascular bed that cause variation of the OCT signal in deeper layers. This reflectance variation will be detected as a flow signal (decorrelation or variance) by OCT angiography algorithms. The artifact is most noticeable in deep reflective structures such as the RPE and can be recognized by the replication of a superficial vascular pattern on the *en face* angiogram of a deeper layer.

Flow Index and Vessel Density

The flow index is calculated as the average decorrelation value (which is correlated with flow velocity) in the selected region. The vessel density is calculated as the percentage area occupied by vessels in the selected region.

Avascular Area

Avascular area is a significant area (larger than the normal gap between capillaries) devoid of flow signal on an *en face* angiogram. On a retinal OCT angiogram of the macula, the foveal avascular zone (FAZ) produces a normal avascular area.

Nonperfusion (Capillary Dropout) Area

Nonperfusion area refers to an avascular area that should normally be vascular. For example, on an OCT angiogram of the macula, any retinal avascular area outside of the FAZ is considered retinal nonperfusion (capillary dropout) area.

Neovascularization Area

Neovascularization area is the sum of pixel areas in a pathologic neovascular net identified on an *en face* OCT angiogram. In proliferative diabetic retinopathy, the area is of vessel growth above the ILM. In age-related macular degeneration, the area is of neovascularization in the outer retina (the region between the outer boundary of the OPL and BM).

REFERENCES

1. Jia Y, *et al.* Split-spectrum amplitude-decorrelation angiography with optical coherence tomography. Opt Express. 2012;20:4710-25.

2. Tokayer J, Jia Y, Dhalla AH, Huang D. Blood flow velocity quantification using split-spectrum amplitude-decorrelation angiography with optical coherence tomography. Biomed Opt Express. 2013;4:1909-24, doi:10.1364/BOE.4.001909 193860 [pii].

Techniques for Using OCT Angiography for Clinical Examination

Tony Ko, Jay Wei

THE ANGIOVUE OCT ANGIOGRAPHY SYSTEM

The AngioVue™ system from Optovue is currently the only commercially available OCT angiography system. It is based on a high-speed (70,000 axial scans per second) SD-OCT platform (RTVue XR Avanti, Optovue Inc.). This chapter will provide practical tips and information on how to best acquire and evaluate clinical OCT angiograms with this system.

PRINCIPLES OF OPERATION

Acquiring an OCT angiogram with AngioVue is as simple as acquiring a traditional three-dimensional OCT volume. Each B-scan in the OCT volume consists of 304 A-scans with each B-scan repeated twice at the same location in order to perform OCT angiography. The entire OCT volume contains 304 B-scans with the resulting OCT angiogram consisting of 304 × 304 pixels. Including the flyback time to return the scan beam to the start of each B-scan, a total of approximately 209,000 A-scans are required to complete the imaging volume. The acquisition time for each AngioVue imaging volume is slightly less than 3 seconds.

The Split-spectrum amplitude decorrelation angiography (SSADA) algorithm is used to detect flowing vessels through the intrinsic motion contrast provided by the flowing erythrocytes.[1] The SSADA algorithm permitted the reduction of the repeated B-scans to the minimum required (two) while still generating high quality OCT angiograms. Involuntary saccades and changes in fixation during data acquisition can lead to motion artifacts that may confound the interpretation of the final OCT angiogram. The AngioVue system uses an orthogonal registration algorithm called "Motion Correction Technology" (MCT) to minimize these motion artifacts[2]. MCT requires the acquisition of a second imaging volume orthogonal in scan direction to the first volume. In AngioVue, the first volume is a horizontal raster (Fast-X) scan while the second volume is a vertical raster (Fast-Y)

scan. Complementary information contained in two orthogonal volumes allows the correction of motion artifacts arising from saccades and small fixation changes.

The motion-corrected OCT angiogram is displayed along with the corresponding OCT intensity en face image and OCT B-scans allowing the direct comparison of OCT structural and functional information. Automatic segmentation of the intra-retinal layers creates 4 default *en face* display windows which are defined here:
- **Superficial capillary plexus**—3 µm below the ILM to 15 µm below IPL
- **Deep capillary plexus**—15 to 70 µm below the IPL
- **Outer retina**—70 µm below the IPL to 30 µm below the RPE reference
- **Choroid capillary**—30 to 60 µm below the RPE reference.

The AngioVue software allows the user to interactively change the boundary definition to each *en face* display windows in order to produce the best visualization of pathologic features.

VESSELS OF THE DEEP CHOROID

The large vessels of the deep choroid have high flow velocity and are characterized by an absence of OCT signal in the B-scan. This is probably due to a combination of OCT signal attenuation from the presence of RPE and choriocapillaris as well as OCT fringe washout from the high flow velocities in the large vessels of the deep choroid. Therefore, OCT signals returning from the vessels of the deep choroid are usually not detected and OCT angiography often cannot be performed in these layers. Vessels of the deep choroid can actually be visualized better using the OCT intensity en face image. Since deep choroidal vessels typically lack OCT signal while the surrounding stroma contains OCT signal, the vessels of the deep choroid will often appear as dark vessels in relief of the surrounding bright stroma in the OCT intensity en face. However, it has been observed that the vessels of the deep choroid can be visualized in OCT angiography underneath areas of geographic atrophy. The absence of RPE and choriocapillaris in these regions likely permits sufficient OCT signals to reach the deep choroid, enabling vessel visualization in the OCT angiogram.

ACQUISITION WORKFLOW

The scan sizes allowed in the Angio Retina scan are 3 × 3, 6 × 6, and 8 × 8 mm while the scan sizes allowed in the Angio Disc scan are 3 × 3 and 4.5 × 4.5 mm. Since all scan sizes are acquired with 304 × 304 A-scans per volume, the smaller scan sizes will produce the highest quality OCT angiograms while larger scan sizes allow wider area coverage to aid multimodality comparisons. By default, all OCT angiography scans use the vitreoretinal (i.e. non-EDI) mode of acquisition to place emphasis on the retinal vessels. Although not recommended, it is possible to change to the chorioretinal (i.e. EDI) mode at this point in the acquisition workflow.

After the acquisition of the each volume, the software will display the OCT angiogram (from all layers) of the just acquired volume. At this point, the patient is allowed to replenish their tear film by either closing or blinking their eyes. The operator should examine the displayed angiogram for evidence of blinks or motion artifacts from fixation loss, beam following, or excessive saccades; the presence of which should necessitate a rescan before continuing to the next acquisition step.

After the completion of the Fast-X and Fast-Y volumes, the software will perform MCT calculations to remove the remaining saccades and minor fixation changes and display the motion-corrected OCT angiogram (from all layers). The operator should examine the final angiogram for evidence that the vessels are well connected and no obvious motion artifacts remain (Fig. 4.1).

UNDERSTANDING MOTION CORRECTION TECHNOLOGY

Motion correction technology (MCT) is best at removing quick involuntary saccades that may occur, for some patients, during the 3 second acquisition window. These saccades are detected by SSADA algorithm as bulk motion (i.e. the entire B-scan is moving) and show up in the OCT angiogram as straight narrow bright lines across the entire image. MCT can be good at correcting the motion artifacts associated with a sufficiently small number of involuntary saccades (typically five or less). MCT will not work well in cases where there is an absence of OCT data from blinking (dark bands in the OCT volume), beam following (image streaks caused by repeating A-scans), or fixation jumping (patches of repeated vessel pattern in the OCT angiogram). The AngioVue software provides an opportunity for the operator to assess the quality of each OCT angiogram for excessive motion before proceeding to the next acquisition step.

The MCT algorithm makes the assumption that the acquisition of the Fast-X and Fast-Y volumes is from the same

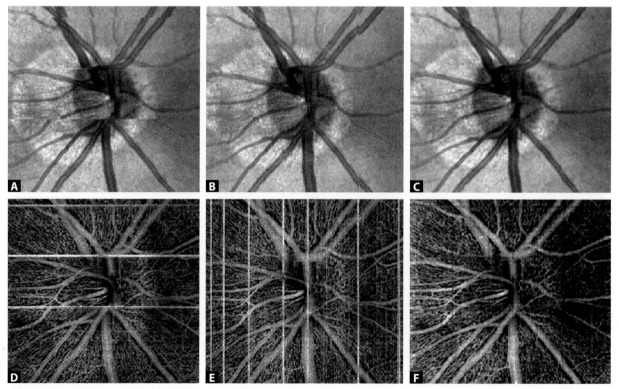

Figs 4.1A to F: OCT intensity en face (A to C) and OCT angiograms (D to F) demonstrating the effect of Motion Correction Technology. Saccadic motion in the Fast-X volume (A, D) are shown as horizontal breaks in the vascular pattern of the intensity en face and straight horizontal lines in the OCT angiogram. Saccadic motion in the Fast-Y volume (B, E) are shown as vertical breaks in the vascular pattern of the intensity en face and straight vertical lines in the OCT angiogram. Motion Correction Technology repairs the breaks in the vascular pattern of the intensity en face image and removes the bright lines from the OCT angiogram (C, F).

anatomical position, so the patient should keep their fixation as close to the same position as possible for both volumes and should not move their head out of the chin rest before the completion of both MCT volumes. If the patient cannot maintain fixation sufficiently well, the MCT algorithm may fail due to the mismatch of anatomic information contained in the two input volumes. In such a case, the AngioVue software provides an option to show only the Fast-X volume by selecting the "No MCT" button to turn off display of the MCT results.

RECOGNIZING ARTIFACTS IN OCT ANGIOGRAPHY

OCT angiography is an OCT-based technique; therefore, any imaging artifact that affects the quality of the OCT B-scan will also affect the quality of the resulting OCT angiogram. For example, floaters can partially obstruct the OCT beam and

cause the A-scans underneath the floater to appear dark in the OCT B-scan. The OCT angiogram in the presence of floaters may also show areas of apparent low perfusion underneath the floater because the OCT signal intensity is low and the apparent OCT angiography signal will also be low. The AngioVue software displays the OCT intensity en face and B-scans along with the OCT angiogram, allowing the user to identify the presence of floaters in the structure OCT images (Fig. 4.2).

Flow projection artifacts occur most strongly at the RPE layer and are caused by the fluctuating shadows cast by the inner retinal vessels. The RPE is a highly reflective layer and the fluctuating OCT signal returning from the RPE cannot be differentiated from true vessels; therefore, the vascular patterns of the inner retina are replicated in the RPE. The AngioVue software provides a tool to suppress flow projection artifacts by subtracting the overlying vessel patterns at the level of the Outer Retina (Fig. 4.3). This can be turned on or off with a "Remove Artifacts" check box.

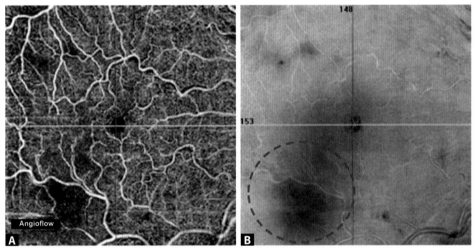

Figs 4.2A and B: A 6 × 6 mm OCT angiogram (A) and the corresponding OCT intensity en face (B) indicating the presence of floaters (dashed red circle) above the imaging volume. The floater partially obstructs the OCT beam and casts dark shadows onto the OCT intensity en face and causes areas of apparent low perfusion in the OCT angiogram. Careful evaluation of both the OCT intensity en face and OCT angiogram is necessary to rule out the image artifacts caused by floaters.

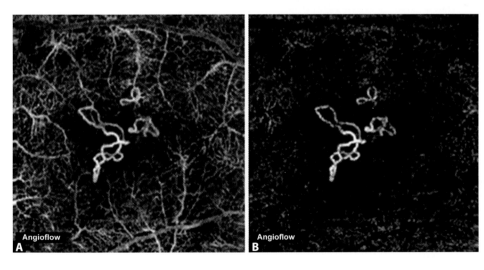

Figs 4.3A and B: OCT angiogram at the level of the outer retina with flow projection artifact from the inner retinal vessels (A) and with flow projection artifact suppressed (B). Flow projection artifact suppression is useful in the visualization of CNV in the outer retina.

REFERENCES

1. Jia Y, Tan O, Tokayer J, et al. Split-spectrum amplitude-decorrelation angiography with optical coherence tomography. Optics Express. 2012; 20:4710.

2. Kraus M, Liu J, et al. Quantitative 3D-OCT motion correction with tilt and illuimnation correction, robust similarity measure and regularization. Biomedical Optics Express. 2014; 5:2591.

Clinical Applications of OCT SSADA Angiography in Everyday Clinical Practice

Bruno Lumbroso, Marco Rispoli, Maria Cristina Savastano

OCT angiography clinical applications can be subdivided into two main categories:

1. Inner retina disorders as retinopathies, vascular acquired or congenital disorders and malformations, and
2. Outer retina and choroidal disorders, mainly choroidal neovascularizations (CNV).

All the figures in this chapter were obtained with a commercial spectral domain OCT device (SD-OCT, XR Avanti "Angiovue", Optovue, Fremont, CA) imaging at 840 nm wavelength. Two automated segmentation lines were manually tuned to be located at desired position. Blood flow between these segmentation lines was registered. An artifact removal function was used to eliminate the retinal vessel shadowing.

INNER RETINA DISORDERS
Age-related Retinal Anomalies

In aged persons, some alterations can be seen at deep vascular plexus level. Angio-OCT shows that the main superficial retinal vessels are normal. At the level of the deep plexus, the capillaries are rarefied. Vessels lose part of their collateral branches. The capillaries have the aspect of irregular fans (Fig. 5.1).

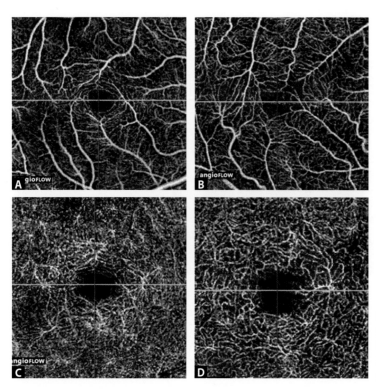

Figs 5.1A to D: (A) Superficial plexus in young man 20 years old. (B) Superficial plexus in man 80 years old man. (C) Deep plexus in young man 20 years old. (D) Deep plexus in man 80 years old man.

Superficial Plexus Anomalies in Macular Pucker

Pucker retinal folds and retraction cause course anomalies at level of the superficial plexus. The vessels lose most of their normal spider net features and mostly follow the folds course (Fig. 5.2).

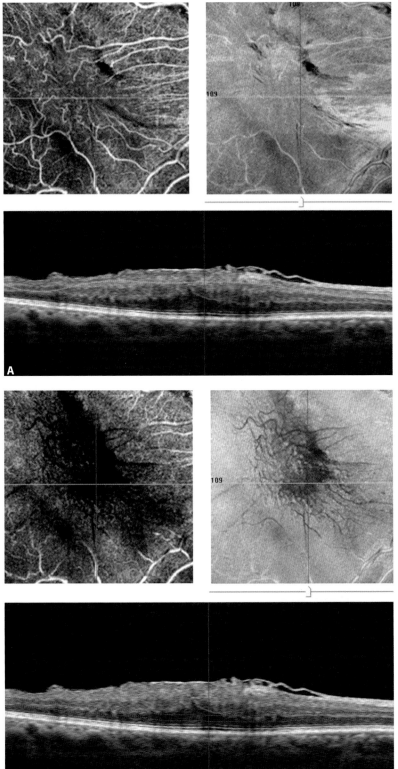

Figs 5.2A and B: (A) Macular pucker: Retinal folds and retraction cause course anomalies at level of the superficial plexus that loses normal spider net features and follows the folds course; (B) Macular Pucker: Deep plexus is difficult to explore due to superficial retinal opacities

Retinal Anomalies and Coat's Disease

Leber Coat's disease presents telangiectasia and aneurysmal vasodilation. In the later stages of the disorder exudates and exudations appear (Fig. 5.3).[1]

OCT angiography shows at the level of the superficial plexus, the vessels lose most of their collateral branches are tangled and present many harmonious shaped loops. The capillaries are rarefied and anomalies in vessel size, vasodilation and macroaneurysms are evident.

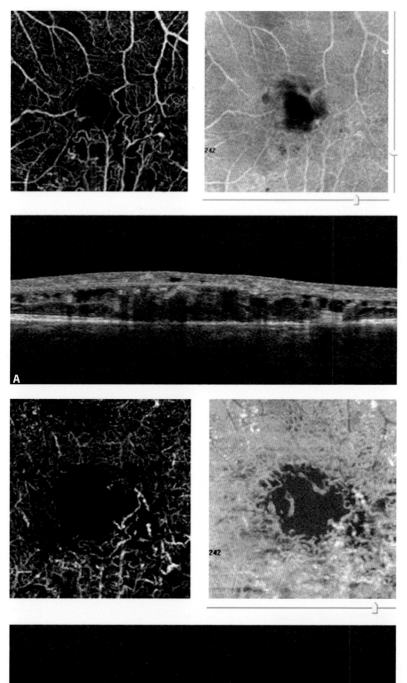

Figs 5.3A and B: (A) Leber Coat's disease: At the superficial plexus, the vessels are tangled and present many loops. The capillaries are rarefied and show anomalies in size, and macroaneurysms are evident; (B) Leber Coat's disease: At deep plexus level capillary drop out is evident, as are size alterations, flow alterations and morphological anomalies with very irregular capillary fans.

At deep plexus level, the capillary dropout is even more evident, as are size alterations, flow alterations and morphological anomalies. The capillary fans are very irregular. Inside the deep vascular net we can see flow anomalies (vasodilation) that are more evident in the deeper levels.

Macular Telangiectasia

Macular telangiectasia shows aneurysmal vasodilation.[2] The main superficial retinal vessels lose most of their collateral branches and present many loops. The capillaries are rarefied and anomalies in vessel size, vasodilation and macroaneurysms

are evident. At deep plexus level, size alterations, flow alterations and morphology anomalies of the plexus are evident. The capillary fans are irregular. Later in evolution exudates and exudations will appear (Fig. 5.4).

Macroaneurysm

OCT angiography shows macroaneurysm as a rounded cavity located in the deep retinal vascular plexus level. It is surrounded by cystoid edema cells. 15 days after laser treatment, the vascular anomaly disappears, and edema cells decrease. Note the star-shaped hard exudates at this retina level (Fig. 5.5).

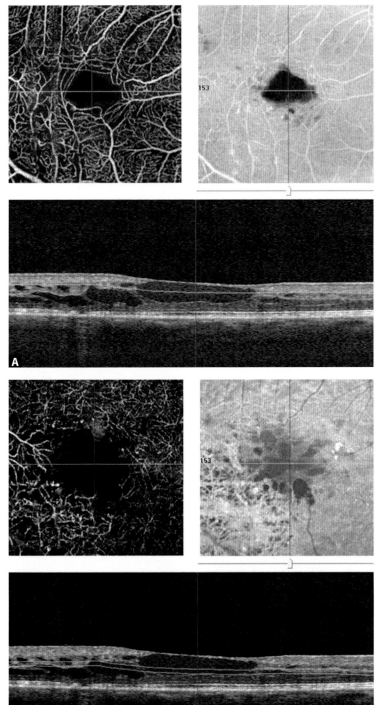

Figs 5.4A and B: (A) Macular telangiectasia. Superficial retinal vessels lose most of their collateral branches and present many loops, capillaries rarefied vasodilation and macroaneurysms; (B) Macular telangiectasia. At deep plexus level, size alterations, flow alterations are evident. The capillary fans are irregular.

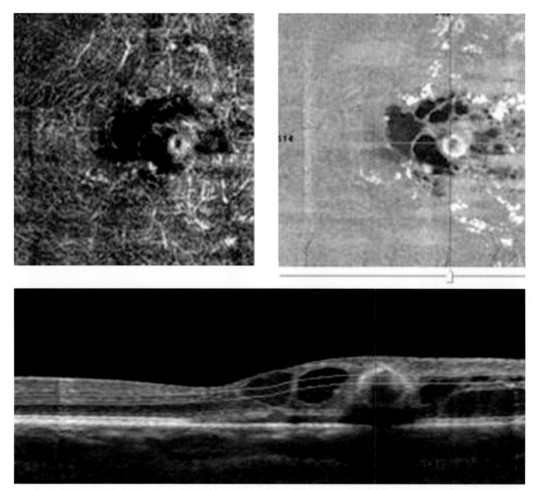

Fig. 5.5: Macroaneurysm: A rounded cavity is surrounded by cystoid edema cells. There are star-shaped hard exudates around the vascular lesion.

Diabetic Retinopathy

Diabetic Patients without Retinopathy: The Avascular Zone

In diabetic patients, even in the absence of retinopathy, angio-OCT shows that the avascular foveal area is larger than in healthy individuals.

A sharp macular capillary network is suggestive of an incipient retinopathy because, even before the onset of diabetic retinopathy, as there are changes in the macular capillary network. The size of some capillaries increases, some are thicker while others are closed and thus we see a looser network with larger and more sparse meshes.

There is an increase in the size of the foveal avascular area that normally is about 500 microns large.[3] This is an early sign that appears before the onset of the microaneurysms and at this stage the condition is still reversible. As retinopathy evolves, the capillary network of the macula becomes increasingly evident and more marked alterations will appear such as mild congestion of capillaries and some dilation. The presence of small non-perfused areas at the posterior pole will lead to the occlusion of small branches; the network becomes at first more irregular, and later, the small areas of ischemia will grow and then merge with the central enlarged avascular area (Fig. 5.6).

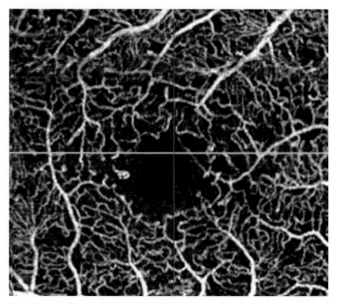

Fig. 5.6: Diabetic retinopathy avascular zone. Increase in the size of the foveal avascular area. This is an early sign that appears before the onset of the diabetic retinopathy and microaneurysms.

Background Diabetic Retinopathy

In patients with background retinopathy, capillary non-perfusion areas, similar to the non-perfused areas, highlighted by fluorangiography, are evident. Angio-OCT shows a larger number of capillary loops and arteriovenous anastomoses. At the level of the deep capillary vascular plexus, the capillary drop out is more evident. Changes in size, in flow and in the morphology of the plexus are evident. Often the scarce capillaries have the shape of a fan. The connections between superficial and deep vascular network are very evident; these are not seen on the fluorangiography. Angio-OCT offers a much better view of shunts, deep connections and vascular loops. The deep new vessels are more clearly seen than with angiography. Rare retinal hemorrhages are visible as masked areas but they are less evident than they appear in fluorangiography (Fig. 5.7).

Angio-OCT does not show up all the microaneurysms: those that are evident are generally the larger microaneurysms where there is probably residual blood flow.

Advanced Diabetic Retinopathy and Retinal Ischemia

The areas of retinal ischemia, examined with angio-OCT are much sharper than as with fluorangiography because there is no masking effect by dye leakage. Details are appreciated that cannot be seen with fluorangiography because hidden by the dye in the intermediate and later stages of the examination.

Ischemic areas show sparse capillaries evident against a grey background. Often the capillaries inside the non-perfusion areas are truncated, with abrupt interruptions, or with shunts. Connections with the deep network are well seen. In angio-OCT the ischemic areas can be easily identified on the basis of texture and of flow alterations (Fig. 5.8).

Initial neovascularizations are seen as thickened and irregular vessels that may emerge from the surface of the retina or from the optic disc.

Proliferative Diabetic Retinopathy

The natural evolution of ischemic area in diabetic retinopathy, or in ischemic venous occlusions, is characterized by the progressive formation of new vessels, preceded by the establishment of capillary shunts, that are clearly visible in fluorangiography immediately after the ischemia appears.[4] With fluorangiography however, it is not possible to appreciate the level of these alterations, but only the two-dimensional course, the veins dilatation and the diffusion of the newly formed capillaries.

In diabetic retinopathy, chronic ischemia leads to proliferative diabetic retinopathy with pre-retinal and pre-papillary neo-vascular membranes. In fluorangiography, there is a very intense dye leakage that does not allow to see the neovascularization.

Angio-OCT of pre-retinal and pre-papillary neovascular membranes allows the operator to make a very precise evaluation of the extent and morphology of the network without the problems linked to dye leakage. Flow and morphology of the neovascular network are visible. Angio OCT can be performed during pregnancy and allows to follow evolution after laser pan retinal photocoagulation (Fig. 5.9).

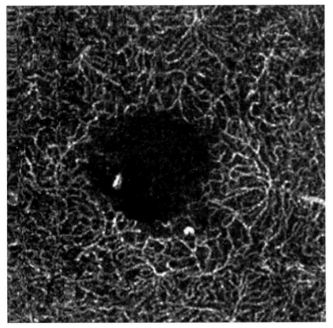

Fig. 5.7: Diabetic retinopathy microaneurysms, enlargement avascular zone. Deep vascular net: Increase in the size of the foveal avascular area and microaneurysms. Vascular fans are irregular.

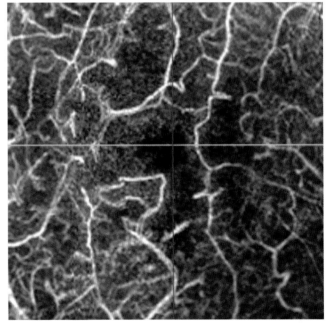

Fig. 5.8: Ischemic areas show sparse capillaries against a gray background. Capillaries inside the non-perfusion areas are truncated, with shunts. Connections with the deep network are well seen.

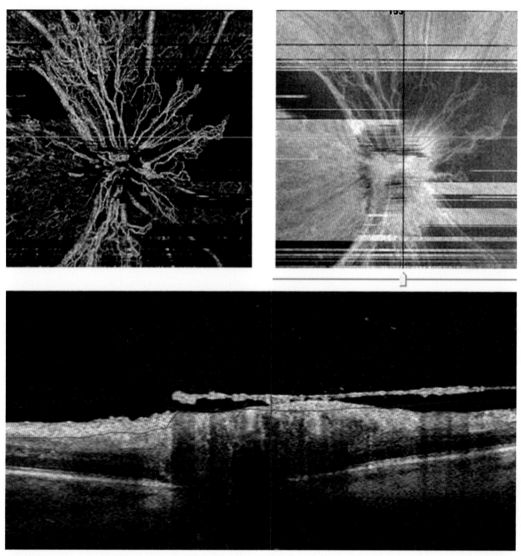

Fig. 5.9: Diabetic proliferative retinopathy angio-OCT in young pregnant woman. Fluorescein angiography could not be performed. Angio-OCT of pre-papillary neovascular membranes allows to make a very precise evaluation of the extent and morphology of the network without any masking by dye leakage. The flow and morphology of the neovascular network are perfectly visible.

Branch Vein Occlusions

In eyes affected by branch vein occlusion, OCT-angiography highlights the vascular network with evident areas of capillary loss that correspond to areas of non-perfusion in fluorangiography. These areas, however, look sharper because there is no masking effect due to dye leakage in intermediate and late stages of the analysis. Some capillaries increases in size while many more are closed. We see thus a looser network with larger and more sparse meshes and a fine, greyish texture (Fig. 5.10).

When the fluorangiography shows staining of the vascular walls the OCT angiography instead shows a very thin vessel (that corresponds to the vessel lumen) surrounded by a darker area that corresponds to the thickened vascular wall. Therefore, there is a sharp visual difference between fluorangiography and angio-OCT.

In vein occlusions, we see changes in the structure of the superficial plexus especially in macular ischemia. The vascular signal (flow) is not linear but has focal deviations, the wall thickness is not regular but shows focal segmentation and lumen narrowing; the vessels course shows abrupt interruptions with some dilation around the avascular foveal area that appears to be widened with respect to healthy individuals. Vessel flow can be segmented. The vascular network is seen more sharply, and the arteriovenous anastomoses and vascular loops are easier to see. We can observe features not seen in fluorangiography because dye leakage hides them in the intermediate and later stages of the examination. Retinal hemorrhages are visible as masked areas but they are much less evident than in fluorangiography.

Retinal edema areas cannot be seen because there is no dye staining. However, in case of edema, we observe a widening and

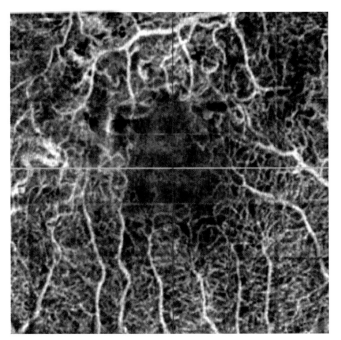

Fig. 5.10: Branch vein occlusion. In the occluded area capillary drop-out is seen, some capillaries increase in size while many more are closed. We see a looser network with larger and more sparse meshes and a fine, greyish texture. Increase in the size of the foveal avascular area.

distortion of the capillary network meshes and a decrease in the sharpness of the widened capillaries.

The deep vascular plexus shows more alteration than the superficial plexus. It varies significantly with considerable differences especially in the ischemic areas. Capillaries distribution is irregular with various changes in vessel course in non-perfused zone. The wall vessels are thicker in the pathologic area; the vessels course shows multiple shunts along various retinal planes.

Branch Artery Occlusion

In case of branch artery occlusion, the superficial vascular network loses some collateral branches (Fig. 5.11A). At deep network level, capillaries of the deep plexus are more affected by the vascular event. Important capillary dropout is evident, some capillaries increase in size while many more are closed. Deep network is loser with larger and more sparse meshes (Fig. 5.11B).

OUTER RETINA DISORDERS
CNV Neovascular Membranes in ARMD

The angio-OCT of neovascular membranes allows the operator to make a very precise evaluation of the extent and morphology of the network without the problems linked to dye leakage or staining.[5] Inside the fibrosis tissue, flow and morphology of the neovascular network are always visible.

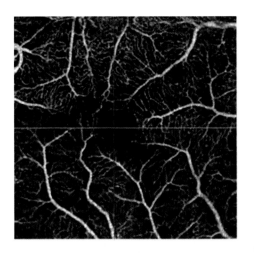

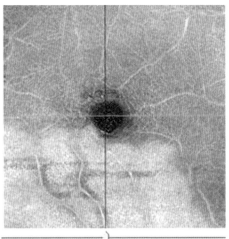

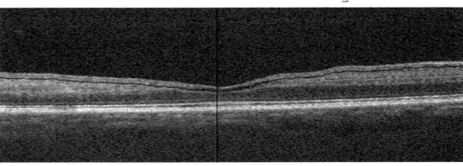

Fig. 5.11A: Branch artery occlusion, superficial network. With angio-OCT, it is possible to highlight the main superficial retinal vessels in the arterial occluded area, that lose some, but not all the collateral branches after the ischemic event. This aspect concerns and the superficial vascular plexus deep before vascular.

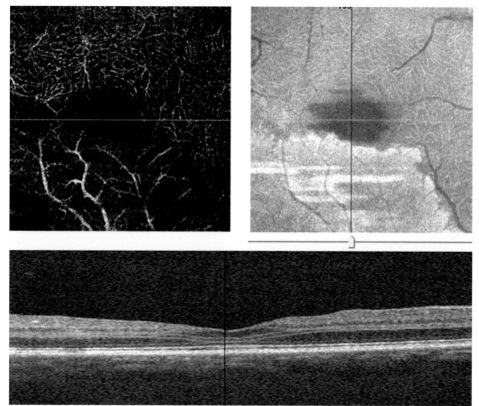

Fig. 5.11B: Branch artery occlusion, deep network. The capillaries of the deep plexus are intensely interested by arterial occlusion. In the occluded area capillary dropout is seen, some capillaries increase in size while many more are closed. We see a wider network with larger and more sparse meshes.

Study of the subretinal neovascularization in fluorangiography provides important data on the progress of the pathology. The new vessels leak the dye, masking rapidly the lesion morphology. The neovascular network is seen only in the early angiographic stages and only for a very few seconds. Following treatment of these lesions with anti-VEGF, it is difficult to precisely observe treatment efficacy because the new vessels stain intensely, even though they could significantly regress. Finally, within a fibrovascular membrane, staining totally masks the neovascular network even when it is greatly reduced by treatment.

Angio-OCT of neovascular membranes allows to be very precise in assessing extent and morphology of the network without the problems linked to the dye. The morphology of the neovascular network inside the fibrovascular formation is always visible. Angio-OCT in the follow-up of intravitreal treatments allows to observe the regression of the new vessels and even their disappearance.

Type 1 CNV

Type 1 CNVs are the more frequently observed new vessels, located below RPE and above Bruch's membrane above the choroid. The new vessels are thin and irregular, inside fibrovascular tissue. Their shape is difficult to define and describe. A feeder trunk can almost or a bunch of feeder vessels are difficult to identify. Anastomoses are irregular. The fluorangiography shows only a diffuse dye leakage. It is very different in the intermediate and late stages because of the almost immediate masking effect produced by dye leakage (Fig. 5.12).

Type 2 CNV

Some neovascular membranes have a tree-like aspect, with fine ramifications that, at times, seem to infiltrate the sub-retinal and retinal tissues. The shape of the new vessels may be similar to a fan, octopus, and spider-web. These vascular flows have irregular features that are totally different from the normal retinal and choroidal vascular networks. New vessels are thin and irregular, at times, located inside non-vascular connective tissue. A feeder trunk can almost always be noticed, or a bunch of feeder vessels, as well as the peripheral anastomoses. Angio-OCT may show the neovascular membranes at times, as cartwheels or bicycle wheels with anastomoses of the peripheral branches that have the peculiarity of being located only within the deep retinal layers above the pigment epithelium (type I2) (Fig. 5.13).

Type 3 CNV

Type 3 CNV are the less frequently observed new vessels, located inside the non-vascular outer retina. They appear as irregular rounded flow formations observed at the level the outer retina layers, at times with a glomerular aspect (Fig. 5.14).

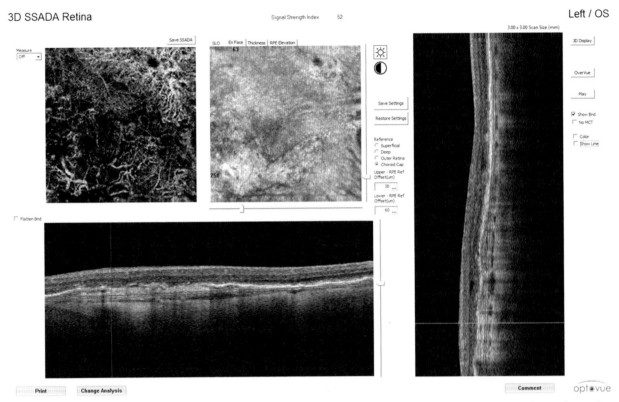

Fig. 5.12: Type 1 CNV located below RPE and above Bruch's membrane above the choroid. The new vessels are thin and irregular. A feeder trunk is present but difficult to identify. Anastomoses are irregular.

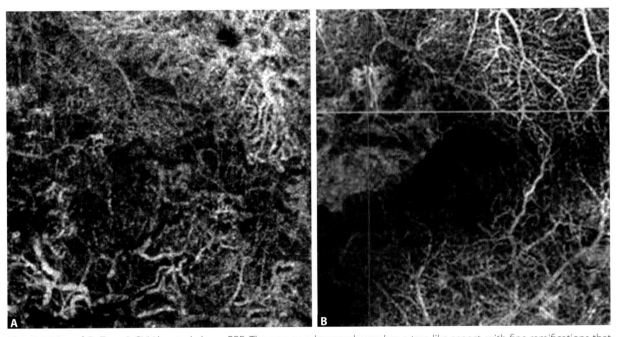

Figs 5.13A and B: Type 2 CNV located above RPE. The neovascular membrane has a tree-like aspect, with fine ramifications that seem to infiltrate the sub-retinal and retinal tissues. New vessels are thin and irregular. A feeder trunk is present but difficult to identify. Anastomoses are irregular.

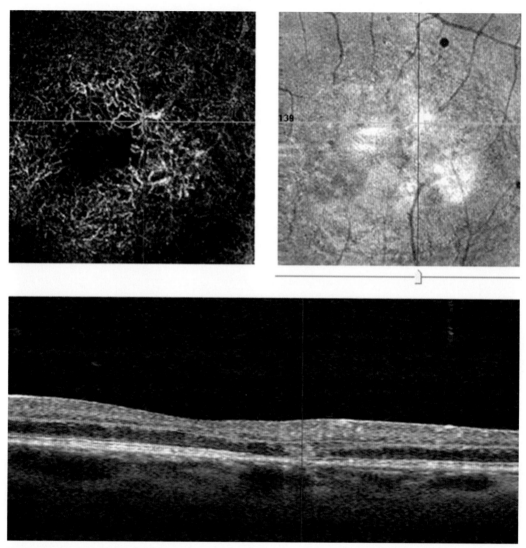

Fig. 5.14: Type 3 CNV located inside the nonvascular outer retina. They appear as irregular rounded flow formations observed with a glomerular aspect. A feeder trunk is present but difficult to identify. Anastomoses are irregular.

CNV Flows in Scars

In the more advanced forms, the angio-OCT shows a small irregular vascular networks inside a capsular formation. The networks are thin and irregular and are observed inside non-vascular tissue. In this case, the OCT horizontal scan will need thickness necessary to detect residual flows inside the fibrosis.

Post-treatment Flows

In our experience the new vessels' apparent regression almost always precedes the reabsorption of the sub-retinal or sub-epithelial fluid and of the edema. In more advanced forms, after repeated treatment, angio-OCT highlights images of small masked vascular networks. The networks are thin and irregular and are observed inside the connective tissue.

In order to obtain a good image, the segmentation will have to include the entire fibrotic area with a thickness sufficient to detect flows inside the thickness of the fibrosis.

After treatment with anti-VEGF, a partial regression of the new vessels can be observed. On the day following the injection of anti-VEGF, many neovascular branches disappear, showing only thinned and sparse residual branches. The vascular network, however, is again visible after seven to ten days. These observations need to be confirmed on a larger number of patients. There are different responses to therapy, due to both the efficacy of the therapeutic substance and the chronic nature of the disorder.

Long-standing Fibrosis

Even in the case of long-standing fibrosis, angio-OCT may provide images of small vascular networks inside the fibrotic scar. We do not know whether these are quiescent new vessels or residual channels, with a minimum amount of blood flow. In old scars, angio-OCT highlights small vascular networks are masked by the fibrous tissue of the fibrotic scar. Segmentation will need a thickness sufficient to detect the flows inside the fibrosis. In some advanced cases, the rarefied capillaries appear to be stable channels.

Neovascular Membranes in Myopic Eyes

Angio-OCT highlights neovascular membranes in myopic eyes as irregular close-knit flow formations observed at the level the deeper retina layers, in contact with RPE. Subretinal myopic new vessels are thin and irregular, at times with a glomerular features. These vascular flows are different from the retinal and choroidal vascular networks. In fluorangiography, their vascular structure is immediately masked by dye leakage (Fig. 5.15).

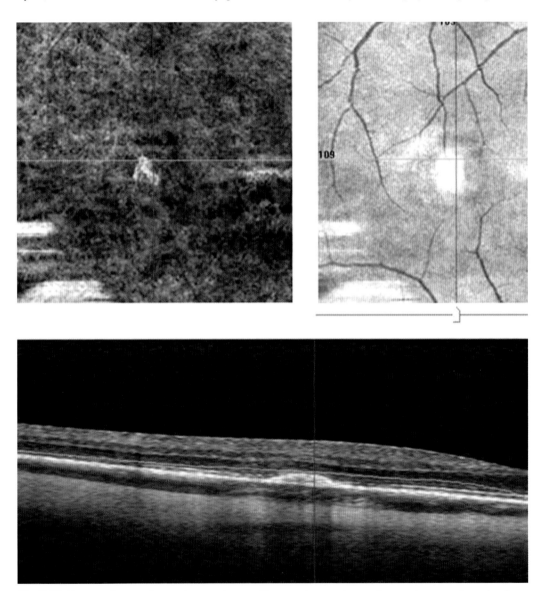

Fig. 5.15: Neovascular membranes in myopic eyes. Neovascular membranes in myopic eyes as irregular close-knit flow formations at the level the deeper retina layers, in contact with RPE. They are thin and irregular, at times with a glomerular aspect.

REFERENCES

1. Jones JH, Kroll AJ, Lou PL, Ryan EA. Coat's disease. Int Ophthalmol Clin. 2001;41:189-98.

2. Yannuzzi LA, Bardal AM, Freund KB, Chen KJ, Eandi CM, Blodi B. Idiopathic macular telangiectasia. 2006. Retina. 2012;32 Suppl 1:450-60.

3. Gariano RF. Special features of human retinal angiogenesis. Eye. 2010;24:401-7.

4. Cheung N, Mitchell P, Wong TY. Diabetic retinopathy. Lancet. 2010;376:124-36.

5. Jia Y, Bailey ST, Wilson DJ, Tan O, et al. Quantitative optical coherence tomography angiography of choroidal neovascularization in age-related macular degeneration. Ophthalmology. 2014;121:1435-44.

Retinal Normal Vascularization

Maria Cristina Savastano, Marco Rispoli, Bruno Lumbroso

With the study of the anatomy of the retina using OCT-angiography we see the histological vascular structure of the retina in vivo without using any dye.[1] In the past, the anatomy could only be seen in histological sections and vessel casts. Understanding OCT-angiography imaging demands in-depth knowledge of histology.

The classical anatomic studies carried out in the first half of the 20th century showed that the distribution of retinal vessels is organized into three distinct layers: 1) superficial plexus, observable with the ophthalmoscope with the large and average sized vessels distributed in the retinal nerve fiber layer; 2) inner plexus, a body of small-sized capillaries located close to the inner surface of the internal nuclear layer; 3) outer plexus: morphologically similar to the internal plexus but located on the outer surface of the external plexiform layer.[2]

OCT-angiography has confirmed these studies in vivo and allows us to study separately the two vascular plexuses, the superficial vascular plexus and the complex internal/external plexus that we have considered as a single deep plexus. The two plexuses clearly have different features that cannot be distinguished by classical fluorescein angiography.[3]

The transition from fluorangiography to OCT-angiography implies a qualitative change in the way images are looked at. At the moment OCT-angiography allows only the study of the posterior pole inside the vascular arcades and the optic disc. We cannot yet, with recent devices, study the retinal periphery beyond the arcade.

All the figures in this chapter were obtained with a commercial spectral domain OCT device, (SD-OCT, XR Avanti "Angiovue", Optovue, Fremont, CA) imaging at 840 nm wavelength. Two automated segmentation lines were manually tuned to be located at desired position. Blood flow between these segmentation lines was registered. An artifact removal function was used to eliminate the retinal vessel shadowing.

ARTERIES AND RETINAL VEINS

The optic disc has a diameter of 1,500 microns while the retinal veins at the edge of the disc have a maximum diameter of around 120 microns. In the mid-periphery the veins have an average diameter of 60 microns. The retinal arteries have a smaller diameter: 80 microns at the edge of the disc, and 50 microns in mid-periphery. In contact with the retinal vessels, in the periarterial avascular area, the capillaries are very rare, virtually absent. Sizes of the arterial and venous capillaries of the retina range between 5 and 10 microns.

THE RETINAL VASCULAR NETWORKS

The sensory retina is supplied with two clearly distinct systems, superficial and deep. Some authors divide the deep plexus in two (inner and outer) nets.

The two parts of the deep plexus cannot be clearly differentiated, since the smaller of 30 micron structures do not have sufficient resolution to give clinically useful imaging. These two parts of the deep plexus will, therefore, be treated here as a single vascular entity, included in a segmentation at the IPL of at least 30 microns.

Superficial Vascular Plexus

Located in the ganglion cell layer and in the nerve fiber layer. The resolution of SSADA OCT-angiography visualizes the superficial vascular plexus with a 60 micron section at the ILM.

Deep Vascular Plexus

Located in the inner nuclear layers and external plexiform. From the anatomical standpoint this plexus consists of two additional nets located respectively on the inside of the inner nuclear and on the outside of the outer plexiform layer. They cannot be individually seen by the OCT-angiography devices and therefore in this chapter we consider them to be a single plexus.

In order to study the two vascular plexuses, we have used specific parameters in the intraretinal level (ILM, IPL, RPE, RPEref), the thickness of the scan being examined and the offset.

Figure 6.1 presents an OCT B-scan with the precise location of the superficial and deep vascular plexus. The superficial plexus is represented by the large retinal vessels located in the innermost layers which measure on average 120 μm. The deep plexus extends between the innermost portion and outer portion of the outer plexiform layer that measures on average around 60 μm.

To assess the superficial plexus, we use a thickness of 60 μm from the ILM to include all the vessels of this plexus.

The parameters for the deep plexus are defined with reference to the IPL in a 30 μm thick scan to visualize the deep plexus in its entirety (Figs 6.2 and 6.3). The two parts of the deep plexus cannot be individually seen by the OCT-angiography, and therefore, we consider them as a single plexus.

OCT-angiography shows that two plexuses have different features.

The superficial plexus features show multiple linear vessels converging towards the fovea and originating from the large upper and lower vascular arcades. Secondary vessels leave the main vessels, forming a web. The thickness of the vessels is homogeneous throughout the length of the scan. The web is grossly regular without vascular meanders or loops. Around the avascular area, the capillaries form continuous peri-foveal arcades with regular meshes.

The deep plexus: Consists of vessels whose orderly pattern distribution around the avascular foveal zone presents interwoven thin horizontal and radial interconnections. The pattern is concentric around the avascular foveal zone. Thickness of the vessels is constant throughout the scan as is their flow.

Connections between superficial and deep nets: The two vascular networks are connected by small slanted interconnection

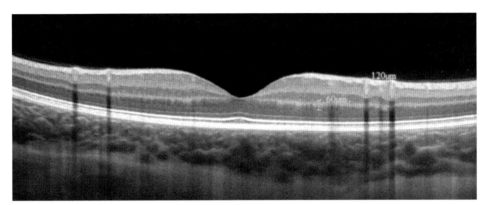

Fig. 6.1: OCT B-scan with location of the superficial and deep vascular plexus. The superficial plexus is represented by large retinal vessels located in the innermost layers whose measurement corresponds on average to 60 μm. The deep plexus extends between the innermost and outer portion of the outer plexiform layer that measures on average about 30 μm.

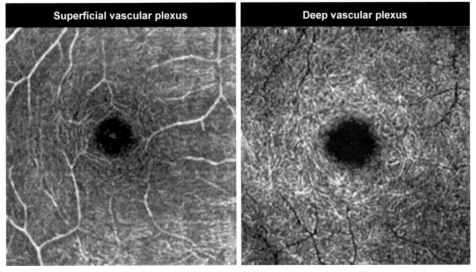

Fig. 6.2: OCT B-scan: The evaluation of the superficial plexus is selected at a thickness of 60 μm from the ILM so as to include all the vessels of this plexus. The parameters for the deep plexus are defined with reference to the IPL in a 30 μm thick scan in order to visualize the deep plexus in its entirety.

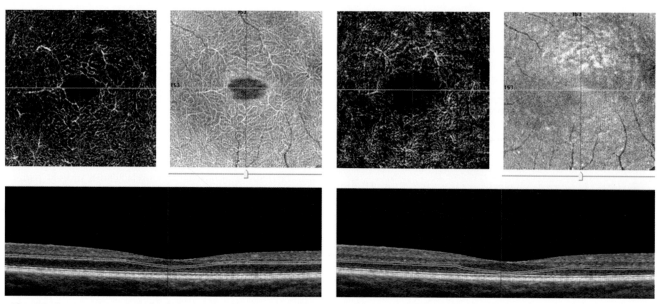

Fig. 6.3: Segmentation superficial plexus: ILM; thickness: 60 micron; Offset: 6 micron. Segmentation deep plexus: IPL; thickness: 30 micron; Offset: OPL level.

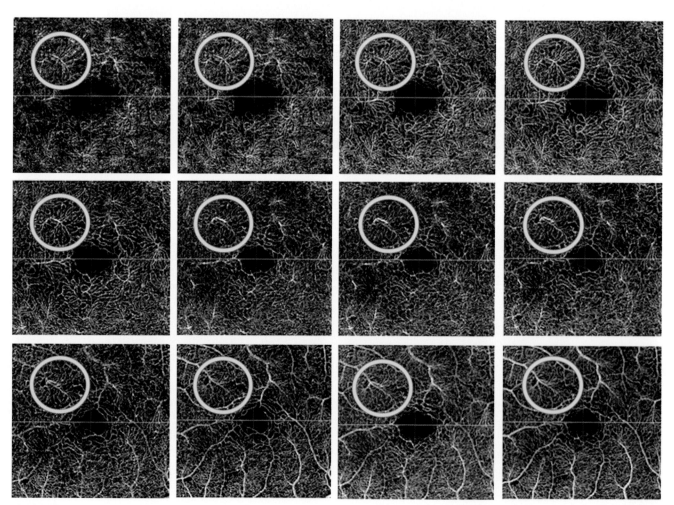

Fig. 6.4: The two vascular networks are connected by small slanted interconnection anastomoses between the superficial and deeper vessels. From the lower extremity of the vertical or diagonal connecting anastomoses horizontal vessels fan out that interconnect to form a complex pattern.[4] This complex pattern is divided in two layers by some authors. In this figure, we show a stack of 16 scans from the deep plexus to the superficial plexus.

anastomoses between the superficial and deeper vessels. From the lower extremity of the vertical or diagonal connecting anastomoses horizontal vessels fan out that interconnect to form a complex pattern.[4] This complex pattern is divided in two layers by some authors (Fig. 6.4).

Avascular foveal zone: Around the avascular area, the capillaries form continuous peri-foveal arcades with regular meshes.

In fluorescein angiography both plexuses overlap and therefore cannot be assessed separately. The overlapping visualization of both plexuses does not make it possible to analyse the superficial and deep vascular features that could be involved separately in some pathological disorders. In healthy eyes, the superficial plexus consists of larger vessels with respect to the deep complex: both plexuses are distributed according to a centripetal pattern around the avascular foveolar zone. The deep plexus consists of small fan-shaped vessels that interconnect to form a complex pattern.

One of the important OCT-angiography limitations is the size of the scan area that involves only the macular region (3×3 mm, 6×6 mm, to 8×8 mm). In the near future a full field will be obtained that will provide further information and offer greater details. Another problem is impossibility to study retina outside the vascular arcades.

REFERENCES

1. Jia Y, Tan O, Tokayer J, et al. Split-spectrum amplitudede correlation angiography with optical coherence tomography. Opt Express 2012;20: 4710–25.

2. Hogan M, Alvarado J, Weddell JE. Histology of the Human Eye—An Atlas and Textbook. Philadelphia: WB Saunders, 1971.

3. Spaide RF, Klancnik JM Jr, Cooney MJ. Retinal vascular layers imaged by fluorescein angiography and optical coherence tomography angiography. JAMA Ophthalmol. 2015;133:45-50.

4. Duke-Elder S. The anatomy of visual system. London 1961;2:372-6.

PART 2

OCT Angiography Study of Diseases and Disorders

Section Outline

Corneal and Anterior Segment OCT Angiography

David Huang, Yan Li, Yali Jia

INTRODUCTION

Optical coherence tomography (OCT) provides higher speed and resolution than other non-contact corneal and anterior segment imaging tests. Commercial available OCT systems, either dedicated to anterior eye imaging (such as Visante or Casia) or hybrid retina/cornea platforms (such as RTVue or Cirrus), have been widely used in managing corneal disease, monitoring anterior angle structure, and planning for anterior eye surgeries.

ANTERIOR SEGMENT OCT ANGIOGRAPHY

Conventional OCT only illustrates the structure information of the bio-tissue. As OCT tecnology advances, the new development of OCT angiography offers a precise visualization of intravasal flow without the injection of contrast agents (such as fluorescein or indocyanine green).[1,2] OCT angiography was initially applied to evaluate posterior segment eye conditions such as retinopathies or choroidal neovascularization.[3, 4] In brief, OCT angiography detects motion caused by moving blood cells or flow. Repeated cross-sectional images (B-scans) at the same scan location were acquired in order to generate motion contrast. If the tissue is stationary, all the pixels will be the same in repeated B-scans. If there is motion between the repeated B-scans due to blood cells or flow, there will be fluctuations in the OCT signal at pixels where the blood vessels are located. These OCT signal fluctuations can be characterized by decorrelation values calculated at each pixel. Performing a series of repeated B-scans covering an area of interest can create volumetric 3-demensional OCT angiography data. Notably, the recent inventing of the split-spectrum amplitude-decorrelation angiography (SSADA) and optical microangiography (OMAG) techniques greatly improved the *in vivo* blood flow detection.[5-7]

In this chapter, we demonstrated OCT angiography in anterior segment of the eye using an ultra-high speed commercial Fourier-domain OCT (Avanti RTVue XR, Optovue Inc., Fremont CA) with a corneal adapter module (CAM). The Avanti OCT operates at an 840 nm working wavelength range and generates 70,000 axial-scans per second. An angio retina scan pattern (2 repeated B-scans at 304 raster positions, each B-scan consisting of 304 axial-scans, 1 horizontal priority plus 1 vertical priority raster scan volumes) was used to image the ocular conjunctiva, sclera, and iris of healthy volunteers. Using the CAM lens, the nominal scan sizes of 3 mm × 3 mm and 6 mm × 6 mm of the angio retina scan pattern correspond to 4.5 mm × 4.5 mm and 9 mm × 9 mm actual scan areas on corneal and anterior segment of the eye, respectively. SSADA technique was used to detect flow and construct angiograms.[6] Software motion correction was applied to reduced eye motion and combine the horizontal and vertical raster scan volumes (RTVue XR software version 2014.2.0.84). The merged SSADA data was downloaded from the Avanti OCT.

Conjunctival and Scleral OCT Angiography

Conjunctival and scleral vasculatures are responsible for supplying oxygen and nutrition to the limbal area. OCT angiography is helpful documenting the vascular patterns in conjunctival and scleral disease. In order to image a wider area on the ocular surface with Avanti OCT (scan depth is approximately 2 mm in tissue), the subject was instructed to look toward the opposite side of the scan. For example, the subject should rotate his/her eye towards the nasal side if the temporal side of the conjunctiva is scanned. A custom software algorithm was used to identify conjunctival and scleral boundaries and generate depth resolved e*n face* conjunctival and episcleral angiograms by maximum flow projection.

The OCT angiograms revealed rich vascular systems in conjunctiva and episclera (Fig. 7.1).

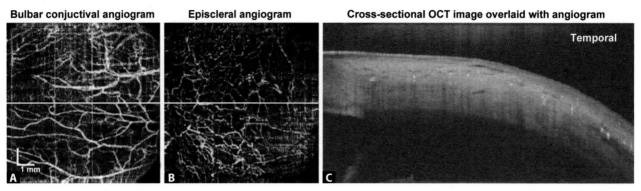

Figs 7.1A to C: *En face* bulbar conjunctival (A) and episcleral (B) OCT angiograms of a human eye. The cross-sectional line scan (C) location was denoted by white lines in (A) and (B). Depth resolved conjunctival (pink) and episcleral (yellow) angiography was overlaid on the cross-sectional OCT structure image.

Iris OCT Angiography

Iris angiography is an important method for examination of disorders of the iris and anterior chamber. Light-colored and dark-colored irises of normal volunteers were imaged with OCT angiography. The subjects were instructed to look straight ahead while OCT images were acquired. The iris angiogram exhibited radial iris vessel patterns in normal light-colored eyes (Fig. 7.2). However, in dark iris the anterior pigment layer produced shadowing and flow artifacts that obscure deeper vasculature (Fig. 7.3).

SUMMARY

Depth-resolved anterior segment OCT angiography can visualize vascular patterns in conjunctiva, sclera and light-colored iris. This technology is potentially useful for the assessment of anterior eye vasculature and local microcirculation.

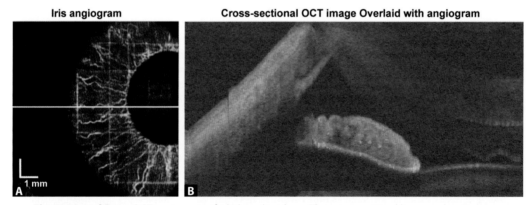

Figs 7.2A and B: Iris OCT angiogram of a light-colored eye. The cross-sectional line scan location was denoted by white lines in (A). The iris angiography (pink) was overlaid on the cross-sectional OCT image.

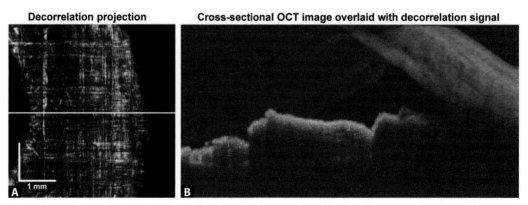

Figs 3A and B: Iris OCT angiographic *en face* projection of a dark-colored eye (A). The cross-sectional line scan (B) location was denoted by white lines in (A).

REFERENCES

1. Makita S, Hong Y, Yamanari M, et al. Optical coherence angiography. Opt Express. 2006;14(17):7821-40.

2. Wang RK, Jacques SL, Ma Z, et al. Three dimensional optical angiography. Opt Express. 2007;15(7):4083-97.

3. Martinet V, Guigui B, Glacet-Bernard A, et al. Macular edema in central retinal vein occlusion: correlation between optical coherence tomography, angiography and visual acuity. Int Ophthalmol. 2012;32(4):369-77.

4. Jia Y, Bailey ST, Wilson DJ, et al. Quantitative optical coherence tomography angiography of choroidal neovascularization in age-related macular degeneration. Ophthalmology. 2014;121(7):1435-44.

5. Li P, An L, Reif R, et al. In vivo microstructural and microvascular imaging of the human corneo-scleral limbus using optical coherence tomography. Biomed Opt Express. 2011;2(11):3109-18.

6. Jia Y, Tan O, Tokayer J, et al. Split-spectrum amplitude-decorrelation angiography with optical coherence tomography. Opt Express. 2012;20(4):4710-25.

7. Choi W, Mohler KJ, Potsaid B, et al. Choriocapillaris and choroidal microvasculature imaging with ultrahigh speed OCT angiography. PLoS One. 2013;8(12):e81499.

OCT Angiography Examination of Choroidal Neovascular Membrane in Exudative Age-related Macular Degeneration

Ching J Chen, Min Wang, Royce Chen, Matthew Olson

INTRODUCTION

Exudative age-related macular degeneration (ARMD) is an advanced form of macular degeneration and is a leading cause of blindness worldwide.[1-3] Exudative ARMD has typically included those patients with distinct choroidal and retinal neovascular membranes, but serous pigment epithelial detachments may also be classified in this category. Vision loss in exudative ARMD occurs secondary to exudation and hemorrhage, in addition to underlying disruption of photoreceptor and retinal pigment epithelial (RPE) architecture.

In 1994, Gass classified choroidal neovascular (CNV) membranes into two distinct categories based on histopathological and fluorescein angiographic features.[4] Green, in 1999, further described the detailed histopathological findings of CNV.[5] Neovascular membranes that were confined to the sub-RPE space were termed Type 1. These membranes often had indistinct borders and corresponded to "occult" leakage patterns on fluorescein angiography. Type 2 neovascularization was characterized by those membranes in which choroidal vessels had penetrated Bruch's membrane and the RPE and had extended into the subretinal space. Angiographically, Type 2 lesions correlated with "classic" leakage patterns, demonstrating early, intense leakage with pooling of fluorescence in the subretinal space.

More recently, Type 3 lesions in exudative ARMD have been characterized.[6,7] This subtype consists of neovascularization extending from the neurosensory retina into the subretinal space and is termed retinal angiomatous proliferation (RAP) lesion. Retinal-choroidal anastomosis may often be demonstrated in advanced cases of Type 3 neovascularization.

Polypoidal choroidal vasculopathy (PCV) is a distinct entity that differs clinically and demographically from neovascular ARMD. These patients have peculiar subretinal polypoidal vascular lesions associated with serous and hemorrhagic retinal pigment epithelial detachment (RPED). The abnormal vasculature changes occur below the RPE.[8-10] This condition is characterized by branching inner choroidal vessels connected to terminal polypoid changes that are located in the macula and peripapillary regions.

Fluoroangiography with fluorescein (FA) and indocyanine green (ICG) dyes have traditionally represented the gold standard in detection and interpretation of vascular changes associated with ARMD.[11-16] Both tests are dynamic two-dimensional studies, and both highlight vessel wall alterations through characteristic fluorescent patterns. FA and ICG are effective in detecting the presence of vascular changes; however, the precise margins and anteroposterior location of pathological vascular lesions often cannot be determined due to obscuration from dye leakage and inability to study the fluoroangiography images in different planes.

Spectral domain optical coherence tomography (SD-OCT) has revolutionized our ability to visualize and understand anatomical changes in the retina and choroid associated with ARMD.[17-21] The combination of high axial resolution, rapid acquisition times, and excellent penetration into the retina and choroid, has provided clinicians with invaluable information about retinal thickening, photoreceptor integrity, and response to therapy. Despite the improved visualization of in vivo retinal and choroidal anatomy, traditional SD-OCT alone has not been able to provide detailed information on retinal and choroidal vasculature.

OCT angiography represents the next major step forward in our ability to both detect and understand the pathogenesis of choroidal neovascular complexes. OCT angiography harnesses the speed and sensitivity of SD-OCT acquisition and pairs it with an amplitude-based algorithm, split-spectrum amplitude-decorrelation angiography (SSADA). This method uses repeated sampling of B scans to allow for detection of decorrelation signals that are resultant from vascular flow.[22,23] OCT angiography, when coupled with en-face OCT imaging, has already proven very powerful in its ability to detect vascular anomalies associated with exudative ARMD and other conditions.[24]

SUBTYPES OF EXUDATIVE AMD AND REPRESENTATIVE CASES

Classification of exudative ARMD is shown in Table 8.1:

TABLE 8.1: Classification of neovascularization in exudative ARMD

Type 1 choroidal neovascularization (Occult)
- Late leakage from undetermined source
- Vascularized retinal pigment epithelial detachment (RPED)
- Sub-RPE space

Type 2 choroidal neovascularization (Classic)
- Subretinal space

Mixed Type 1 and 2 choroidal neovascularization

Type 3 neovascularization: Retinal Angiomatous Proliferation (RAP)

Polypoidal Choroidal Vasculopathy (PCV)

Type 1 Neovascularization

Type 1 neovascularization corresponds to "occult" CNV on fluorescein angiography. Abnormal vessels develop in the choroid and proliferate anteriorly into the sub-RPE space. Fluorescein angiography demonstrates irregular low-grade leakage with stippled hyperfluorescence and late staining (Figs 8.1 to 8.3)

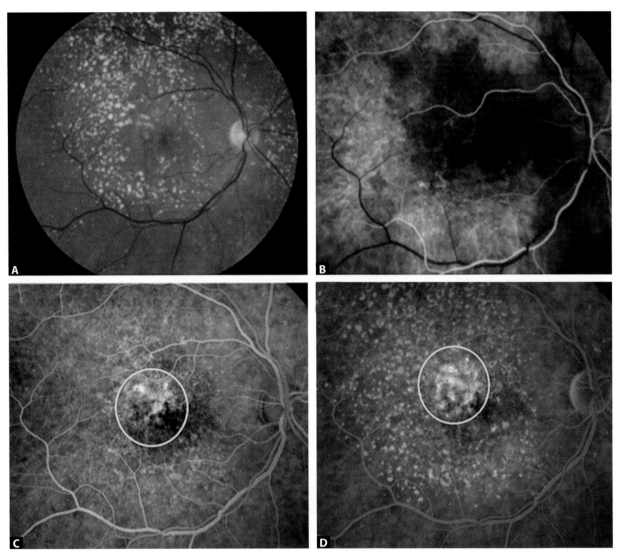

Figs 8.1A to D: Type 1 CNV with late fluorescein oozing from an undetermined source. (A) Color fundus photo shows multiple drusen with some pigmentary change. No subretinal fluid, exudate or hemorrhage is apparent. (B) Arterial phase FA. (C) Early venous phase FA demonstrates fluorescein uptake by the drusen and an area of hyperfluorescence with low grade oozing. (D) Late venous phase FA shows slight increased hyperfluorescence in the same area without a well-defined net.

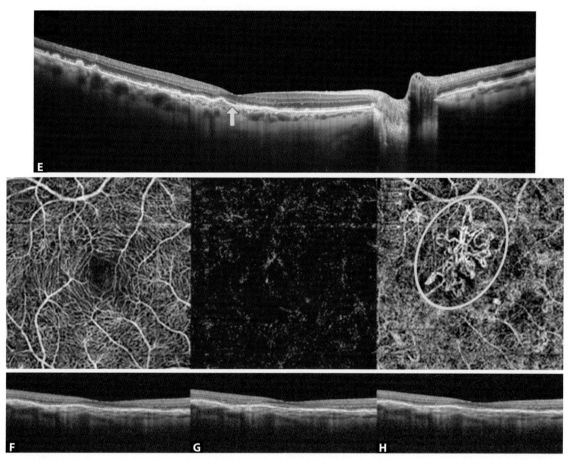

Figs 8.1E to H: Type 1 CNV with late fluorescein oozing from an undetermined source. (E) SD-OCT shows irregularity of RPE and ellipsoid zone with drusen. Mild subretinal fluid is present (yellow arrow). (F) OCT angiography with manual full thickness retinal segmentation shows no abnormal vessels in the outer retina. (G) OCT angiography with manual segmentation by moving the lower border of "default outer retina slab setting" up to the RPE to avoid picking up flow signal from beneath the RPE. No CNV is detected above the RPE. (H) OCT angiography of the choroid slab clearly demonstrates blood flow in a neovascular net. (Red and green colored lines delineate the segmentation plane for each OCT angiography image).

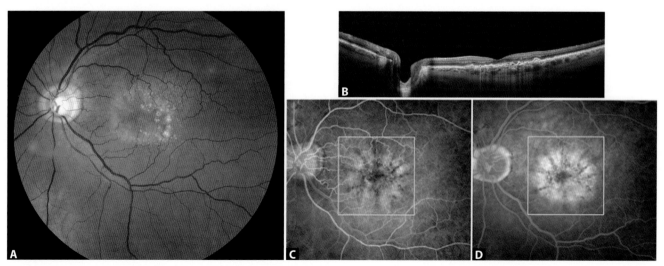

Figs 8.2A to D: Type 1 CNV poorly identified by FA. (A) Color fundus photo shows multiple small to medium size drusen with pigment stippling. Radiating petalloid RPE atrophy is also noted. (B) SD-OCT reveals multiple drusen with irregularity of the RPE and the ellipsoid zone. A small amount of subfoveal fluid is present. (C) Early venous phase FA demonstrates a pigment window defect and some fluorescein staining of drusen. No definite leakage is present. (D) Late venous phase FA: slight increased fluorescence of the area with radiating petalloid pigment atrophy. There is no definite leakage to confirm a CNV.

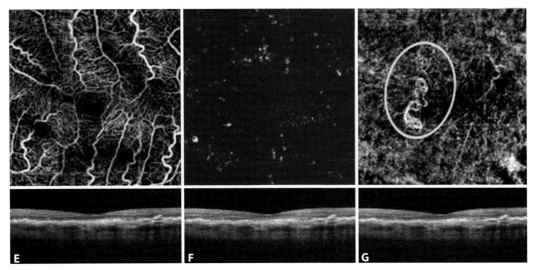

Figs 8.2E to G: Type 1 CNV poorly identified by FA. (E) OCT angiography of the superficial retina slab. No abnormal vessels are present in this section. (F) OCT angiography with manual segmentation by moving the lower border of "default outer retina slab setting" up to the RPE to avoid picking up flow signal below the RPE. No definite CNV is detected. (G) OCT angiography of the choroid slab demonstrates the small, multi-looped CNV (in yellow circle).

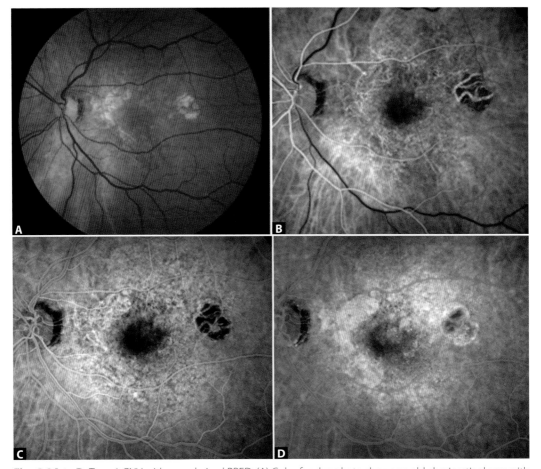

Figs 8.3A to D: Type 1 CNV with vascularized RPED. (A) Color fundus photo shows an old chorioretinal scar with RPE atrophy temporal to the macula. No significant drusen or geographic atrophy are present. The foveal reflex is absent. No classic RPED with well demarcated border can be demonstrated. (B) Arterial phase FA shows pigment window defect corresponding to the chorioretinal scar. There is irregular increased transmission of choroidal fluorescence surrounding the fovea. (C) AV phase FA shows no definite dye pooling or leakage. An extensive irregular pigment window defect is present in the macular area. (D) Late venous phase FA shows faint fluorescein dye pooling temporal to the fovea in addition to the pigment window defect with hyperfluorescence.

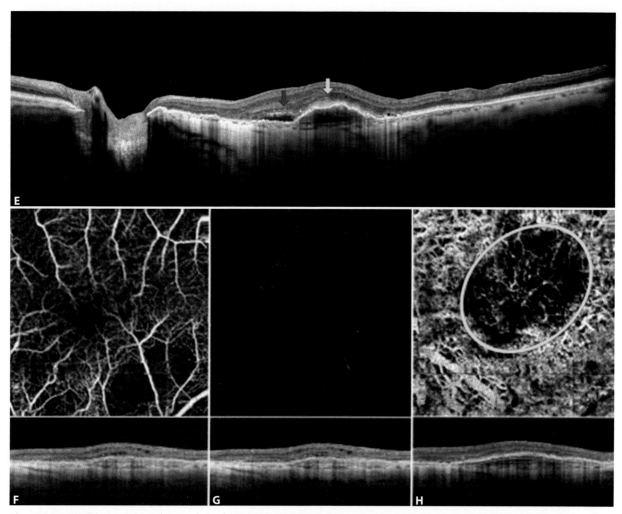

Figs 8.3E to H: Type 1 CNV with vascularized RPED. (E) SD-OCT demonstrates moderately elevated RPED with irregular surface, and some mild hyper-reflective spots adherent to the inner surface of the dome-shaped RPED (yellow arrow). A significant amount of subretinal fluid is present (red arrow). (F) OCT angiography with manual full thickness retinal segmentation shows no abnormal blood flow from the inner retina to the inner RPE surface. (G) Manual segmentation of OCT angiography with a curved reference line at the outer retina above the RPE (green segmentation lines) shows no detectable blood flow. (H) Manual segmentation of OCT angiography with a curved reference line under the dome of the RPED reveals a tree-branch like CNV underneath the RPE (in yellow circle).

Type 2 Neovascularization

Type 2 neovascularization corresponds to "classic" CNV on fluorescein angiography. Abnormal vessels develop in the choroid and proliferate anteriorly, perforating the RPE and extending into the subretinal space. Fluorescein angiography demonstrates early, lacy hyperfluorescence, with late pooling of dye into the subretinal space (Figs 8.4 and 8.5).

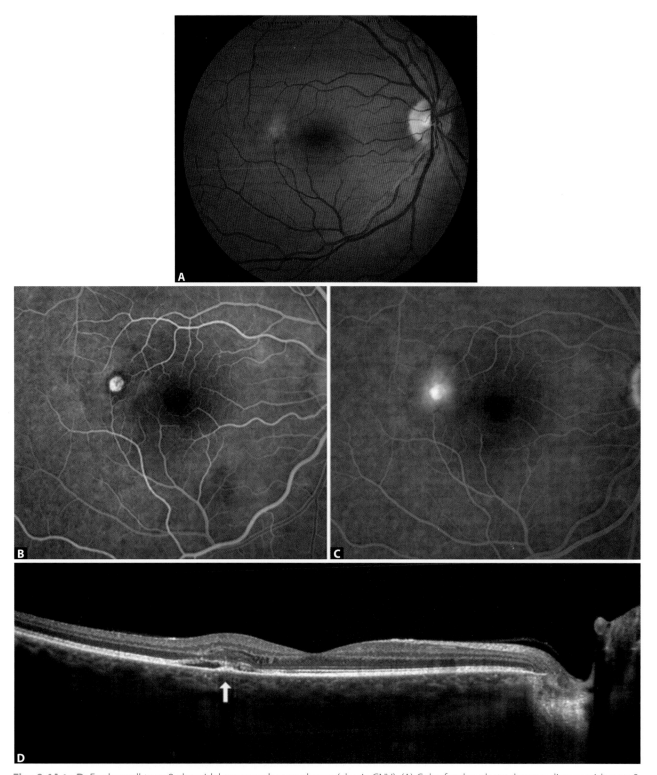

Figs 8.4A to D: Fresh small type 2 choroidal neovascular membrane (classic CNV). (A) Color fundus photo shows a dirty grayish type 2 CNV with adjacent subretinal hemorrhage and surrounding retinal edema. (B) Early venous phase FA at 23 seconds shows a lacy pattern fluorescein filling of the small CNV temporal to the macula with surrounding blocked fluorescence. (C) Late phase FA at 6 minutes and 22 seconds demonstrates intense leakage from the CNV. (D) SD-OCT demonstrates a small subretinal CNV (white arrow) and subretinal fluid.

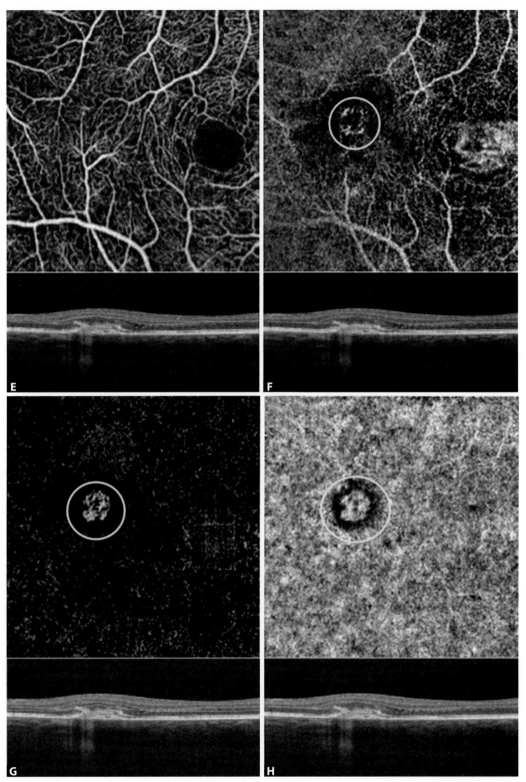

Figs 8.4E to H: Fresh small type 2 choroidal neovascular membrane (classic CNV). (E) Superficial retina slab of the OCT angiography shows no abnormal vascular flow. (F) Manual OCT angiography segmentation with the lower border of tissue slab set just above the RPE and the segmentation thickness reduced to 20 μm, without signal suppresion, shows a small subretinal CNV. (G) OCT angiography of the outer retina and RPE slab shows a significant flow signal from the CNV. (H) OCT angiography of the choroid slab shows the CNV as well. A 360 degree dark zone surrounds the CNV net, corresponding well to the area of blocked fluorescence in FA.

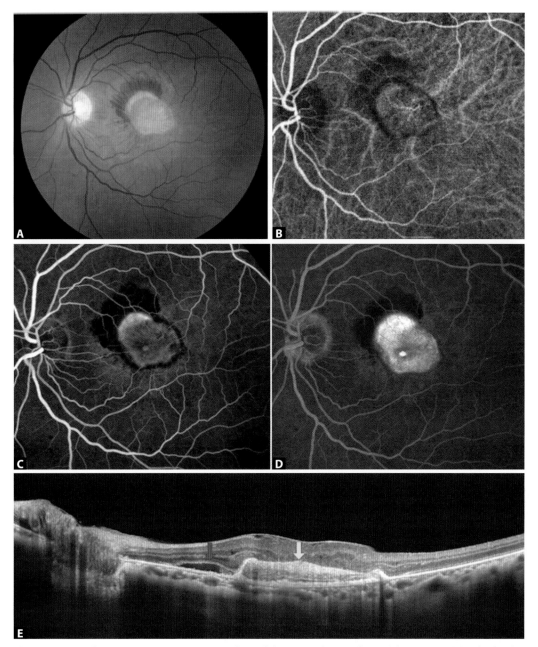

Figs 8.5A to E: Chronic treatment naïve type 2 choroidal neovascular membrane (Classic CNV). (A) Color fundus photo shows a thick fibrovascular CNV and significant subretinal fluid surrounding the CNV complex. Subretinal hemorrhage at the upper border of the CNV complex is also present. (B) ICG angiography confirms a CNV with feeder vessel with surrounding blocked fluorescence. (C) Venous phase FA reveals a bicycle wheel-shaped CNV with fluorescein leakage. There is fluorescein blockage surrounding the CNV. (D) Late phase FA shows fluorescein leakage from CNV with complete staining of the whole complex. The subretinal blood at the upper border of the CNV is causing significant fluorescein blockage. (E) SD-OCT demonstrates a thick fibrovascular membrane under the sensory retina and RPE (yellow arrow). Significant subretinal fluid is present nasal to the fibrovascular membrane (red arrow). Retinal architecture, especially the outer retina in the macular area, is distorted.

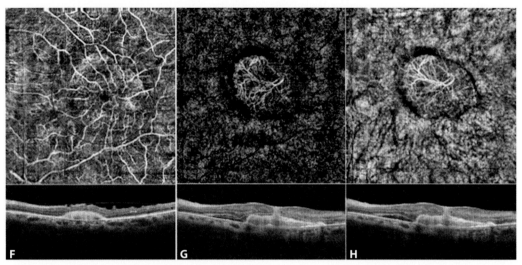

Figs 8.5F to H: Chronic treatment naïve type 2 choroidal neovascular membrane (Classic CNV). (F) OCT angiography with manual full-thickness retinal segmentation demonstrates a see-through large CNV net with significant blood flow. (G) OCT angiography using the default outer retina, RPE slab and signal supression shows a large CNV with multiple branches. (H) OCT angiography of the choroid slab shows signficant blood flow in the thick CNV. A feeder vessel is visible centrally. A 360 degree dark zone surrounds the CNV net, corresponding well to the area of blocked fluorescence in FA.

Mixed Type Neovascularization

Many CNVMs in exudative AMD represent combinations of type 1 and type 2 neovascularization. These lesions accordingly demonstrate features of both "occult" and "classic" CNV on fluorescein angiography (Fig. 8.6).

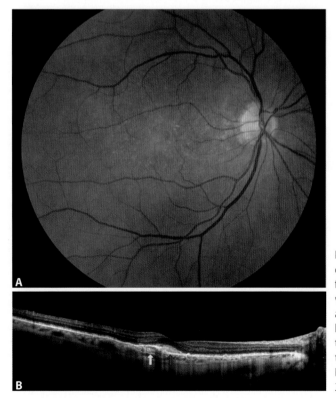

Figs 8.6A and B: Mixed type 1 and type 2 choroidal neovascular membrane. (A) Color fundus photo shows a dirty gray membrane with surroundiing edema in the macular area. (B) SD-OCT shows a type 2 CNV with hyperreflectivity under the central fovea in the subretinal space (red arrow). There is a type 1 CNV with hyper-reflectivity in the sub-RPE space just temporal to the subfoveal type 2 CNV (yellow arrow).

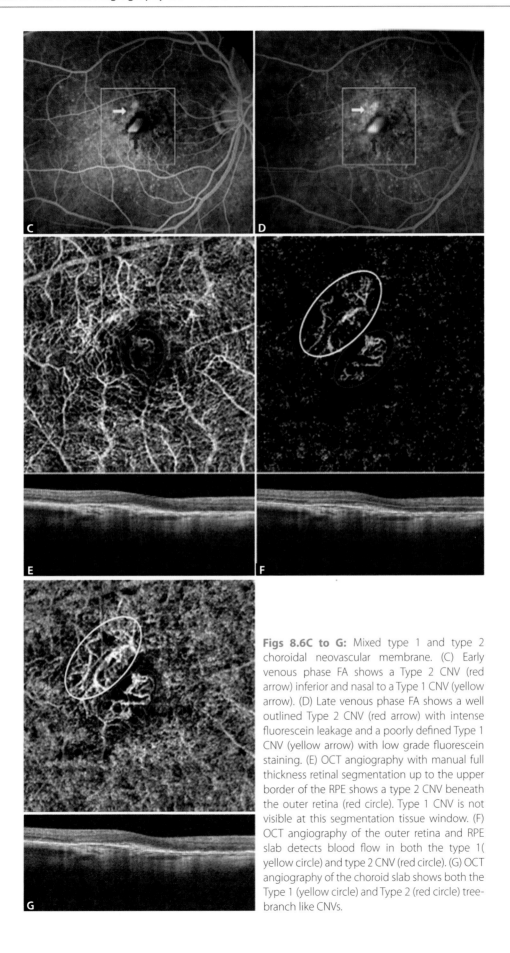

Figs 8.6C to G: Mixed type 1 and type 2 choroidal neovascular membrane. (C) Early venous phase FA shows a Type 2 CNV (red arrow) inferior and nasal to a Type 1 CNV (yellow arrow). (D) Late venous phase FA shows a well outlined Type 2 CNV (red arrow) with intense fluorescein leakage and a poorly defined Type 1 CNV (yellow arrow) with low grade fluorescein staining. (E) OCT angiography with manual full thickness retinal segmentation up to the upper border of the RPE shows a type 2 CNV beneath the outer retina (red circle). Type 1 CNV is not visible at this segmentation tissue window. (F) OCT angiography of the outer retina and RPE slab detects blood flow in both the type 1(yellow circle) and type 2 CNV (red circle). (G) OCT angiography of the choroid slab shows both the Type 1 (yellow circle) and Type 2 (red circle) tree-branch like CNVs.

Type 3 Neovascularization (Retinal Angiomatous Proliferation)

Type 3 neovascularization (RAP lesion) is defined by neovascularization extending from the neurosensory retina. A compensatory intraretinal telangiectatic response occurs, and a feeder arteriole and draining venule are often seen. Retinal-choroidal anastomoses are often present. Fluorescein angiography typically demonstrates early hyperfluorescent "hot spots" with later leakage of dye around these areas (Fig. 8.7).

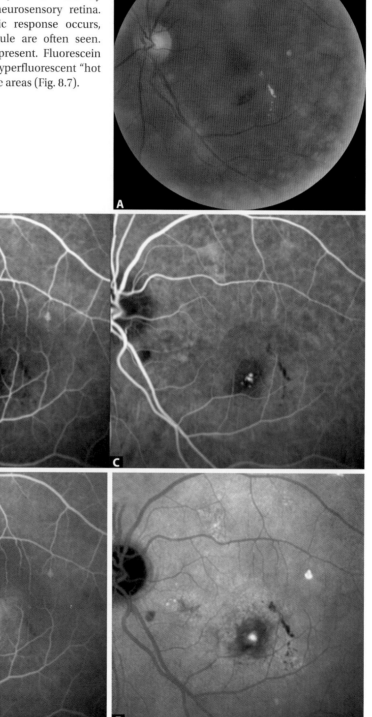

Figs 8.7A to E: Type 3 neovascular membrane (Retinal Angiomatous Proliferation). (A) Color fundus photo shows intraretinal hemorrhage, exudate and retinal edema below the fovea. (B) Simultaneous FA (C) and ICGA at the early phase (1:12.31) show hyperfluorescent spots in the macula. (D) Simultaneous FA and ICGA in the late phase (28:53.56) demonstrate dye leakage on FA and (E) an enlarged hyperfluorescent spot on ICGA surrounded by a hypofluorescent ring in the macula.

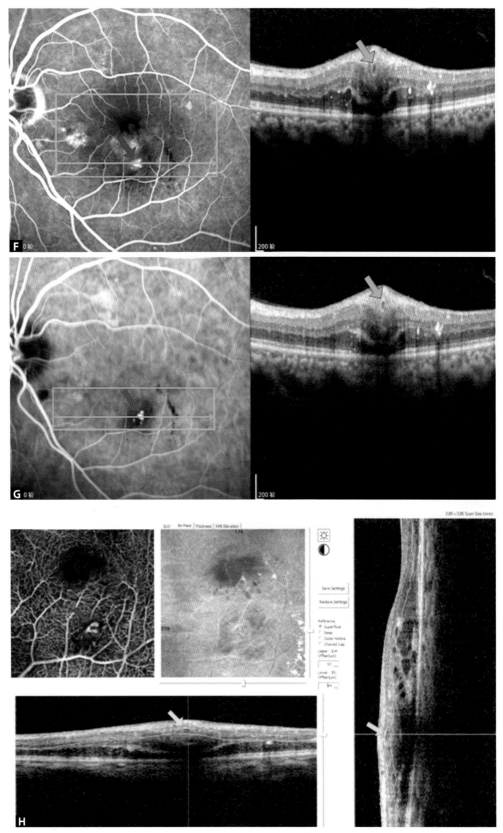

Figs 8.7F to H: Type 3 neovascular membrane (Retinal Angiomatous Proliferation). (F) Simultaneous FA and SD-OCT show a hyperfluorescent spot (red arrow) and a proliferative intraretinal capillary in the inner retina (blue arrow). (G) Simultaneous ICGA and SD-OCT show a hyper-fluorescent spot (red arrow) and proliferative intraretinal capillary in the inner retina (blue arrow). (H) OCT angiography of the deep retina slab shows an enlarged proliferative intraretinal capillary (red arrow) corresponding to the capillary location on SD-OCT (yellow arrows).

Polypoidal Choroidal Vasculopathy

Polypoidal choroidal vasculopathy (PCV) is a distinct entity that differs clinically and demographically from neovascular ARMD. These patients have subretinal polypoidal lesions associated with serous and hemorrhagic RPED. Choroidal vascular channels are connected in a vascular network with terminal polypoid dilations that are commonly found in the macula and peripapillary regions. ICGA is more effective than FA in visualizing the margins and extent of these lesions. Pigment epithelial detachments and associated hemorrhages are frequently encountered (Figs 8.8 and 8.9).

CONCLUSION

Our understanding of the pathological sequences in exudative AMD has been aided greatly by first fluoroangiography, then OCT, and now OCT angiography. Although studies with OCT angiography are currently more limited in acquisition area compared to FA and ICGA, OCT angiography provides non-invasive structural information that often captures greater detail than fluoroangiography studies and OCT alone. In some instances, OCT angiography can reveal pathological vascular changes that may not otherwise be detected.

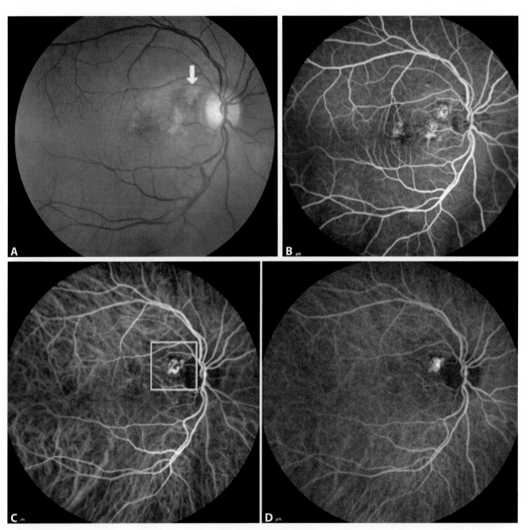

Figs 8.8A to D: Polypoidal Choroidal Vasculopathy (PCV) in a 74-year-old female African-American patient. (A) Color fundus photo shows an orange colored polypoid lesion with small RPED in the peripapillary region with adjacent retinal color changes. (B) FA shows a polypoidal lesion with fluorescein staining. A branch vascular network (BVN) is present adjacent to the polypoidal lesion with mild fluorescein leakage. (C and D) Early and late ICG angiography shows the polypoidal lesion with ICG filling.

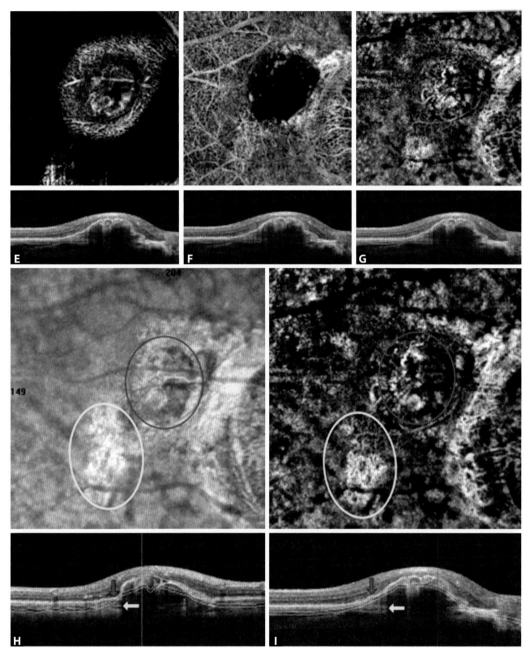

Figs 8.8E to I: Polypoidal Choroidal Vasculopathy (PCV) in a 74-year-old female African-American patient. (E) OCT angiography with a straight segmentation line near the apex of the RPED demonstrates the polypoidal lesion. (F) OCT angiography with a straight segmentation line near the base of the RPED shows some flow signal from the BVN. (G) OCT angiography with a curved segmentation line captures both the polypoidal lesion and BVN. *En face* OCT (H), and OCT angiography (I) segmentation with a curved reference line (green lines) show the polypoidal lesion at the apex of the RPED (red circle) and the BVN (yellow circle) between the RPE (red arrow) and Bruch's membrane (yellow arrow).

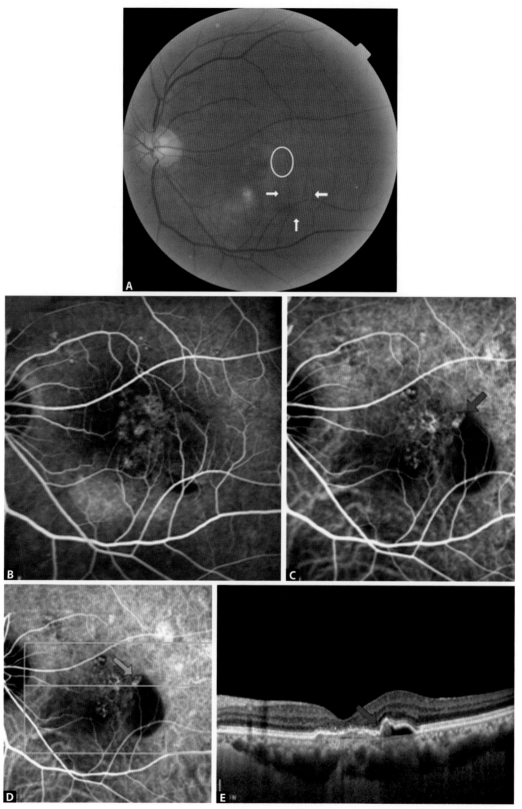

Figs 8.9A to E: Polypoidal choroidal vasculopathy (PCV) in a 62-year-old male Chinese patient. (A) Color fundus photo shows an orange-reddish lesion (yellow circle) and an RPED (white arrows) in the macula. (B and C) Simultaneous FA (B) and ICGA (C) in the early phase (0:43.28) show a polypoidal lesion (red arrow). A branch vascular network is present on the left side of the polypoidal lesion. (D and E) Simultaneous ICGA (1:52.79) and SD-OCT demonstrate the RPED (red arrow) corresponding to the polypoidal lesion (blue arrow).

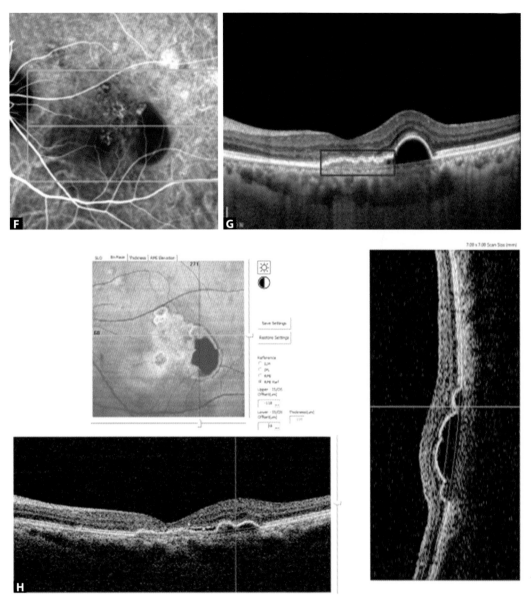

Figs 8.9F to H: Polypoidal choroidal vasculopathy (PCV) in a 62-year-old male Chinese patient. (F and G) SD-OCT (G) reveals the double layer sign (red rectangle) corresponding to the branch vascular network on simultaneous ICGA (F) at 1:52.79). (H): *En face* OCT demonstrates multiple RPEDs with accumulated fluid and clear margins. A branch vascular network on *en face* imaging is present as a hyperreflective area.

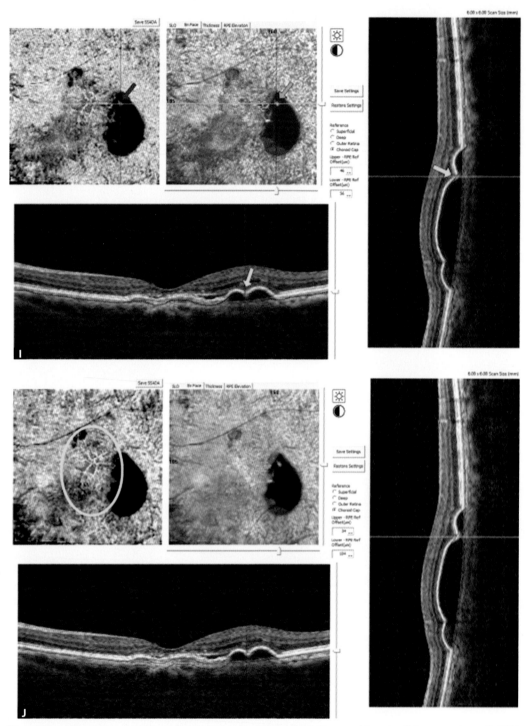

Figs 8.9I and J: Polypoidal Choroidal Vasculopathy (PCV) in a 62-year-old male Chinese patient. (I) OCT angiography and *en face* OCT identified the polypoidal lesion (red and blue arrows) corresponding to the notch (yellow arrows) of RPED on SD-OCT. (J) BVN (yellow circle) is revealed on OCT angiography when the segmentation slab is selected between the RPE and Bruch's membrane.

REFERENCES

1. Klein R, Klein BE, Linton KL. Prevalence of age-related maculopathy. The Beaver Dam Eye Study. Ophthalmology. 1992;99: 933-43.

2. Klein R, Klein BE, Tomany SC, et al. Ten-year incidence and progression of age-related maculopathy: The Beaver Dam Eye Study. Ophthalmology. 2002;109:1767-79.

3. Friedman DS, O'Colmain BJ, Munoz B, et al. Prevalence of age-related macular degeneration in the United States. Arch Ophthalmol. 2004; 122(4): 564-72.

4. Gass JD. Biomicroscopic and histopathologic considerations regarding the feasibility of surgical excision of subfoveal neovascular membranes. Am J Ophthalmol. 1994;118:285-98.

5. Green WR. Histopathology of age-related macular degeneration. Molecular Vision. 1999; 5:27.

6. Yannuzzi LA, Negrão S, Lida T, et al. Retinal angiomatous proliferation in age-related macular degeneration. Retina. 2001;21(5):416-34.

7. Freund KB, Ho IV, Barbazetto IA, Koizumi H, et al. Type 3 neovascularization: the expanded spectrum of retinal angiomatous proliferation. Retina. 2008;28:201-11. doi: 10.1097/IAE.0b013e3181669504.

8. Yannuzzi L, Sorenson J, Spaide RF, Lipson B. Idiopathic polypoidal choroidal vasculopathy. Retina. 1990;10:1-8.

9. Yannuzzi LA, Wong DWK, Sforzolini BS, et al. Polypoidal choroidal vasculopathy and neovascularized age-related macular degeneration. Arch Ophthalmol. 1999;117(11):1503-01.

10. Sho K, Takahashi K, Yamada H, et al. Polypoidal choroidal vasculopathy: incidence, demographic features, and clinical characteristics. Arch Ophthalmol. 2003;121(10):1392-6.

11. Olsen TW, Feng X, Kasper TJ. Fluorescein angiographic lesion type frequency in neovascular age-related macular degeneration. Ophthalmology. 2004;111(2):250-5.

12. Soubrane G, Coscas G, França C, et al. Occult subretinal new vessels in age-related macular degeneration. Natural history and early laser treatment. Ophthalmology. 1990;97(5):649-57.

13. Jorzik JJ, Almut B, Stefan D, et al. Digital simultaneous fluorescein and indocyanine green angiography, autofluorescence, and red-free imaging with a solid state laser-based confocal scanning laser ophthalmoscope. Retina. 2005;25(4):405-16.

14. Guyer DR, Yannuzzi LA, Slakter JS, et al. Digital indocyanine-green videoangiography of occult choroidal neovascularization. Ophthalmology. 1994;101(10):1727-37.

15. Regilio CD, Benson WE, Maguire JI, et al. Indocyanine green angiography and occult choroidal neovascularization. Ophthalmology. 1994;101(2):280-8.

16. Guyer DR, Yannuzzi LA, Slakter JS. Classification of choroidal neovascularization by digital indocyanine green angiography. Ophthalmology. 1996;103(12):2054-60.

17. Hee MR, Baumal CR, Puliafito CA, et al. Optical coherence tomography of age-related macular degeneration and choroidal neovascularization. Ophthalmology. 1996;103(8):1260-70.

18. Coscas F, Coscas G, Souied E, et al. Optical coherence tomography identification of occult choroidal neovascularization in age-related macular degeneration. Am J Ophthalmol. 2007;144(4):592-9.

19. Gess AJ, Fung AE, Rodriquez JG. Imaging in neovascular age-related macular degeneration. Semin Ophthalmol. 2011;26:225-33.

20. Schmidt-Erfurth U, Chong V, Loewenstein A, et al. Guidelines for the management of neovascular are-related macular degeneration by the European Society of Retina Specialists (EURETINA). Br J Ophthalmol. 2014; 98:1144-67.

21. Mathew R, Pefkianaki M, Kopsachilis N, et al. Correlation of fundus fluorescein angiography and spectral domain optical coherence tomography in identification of membrane subtypes in neovascular arge-related macular degeneration. Ophthalmologica. 2014;231: 153-9.

22. Jia Y, Tan O, Tokayer J, Potsaid B, Wang Y, Liu JJ, et al. Split-spectrum amplitude-decorrelation angiography with optical coherence tomography. Opt Express. 2012;20:4710-24.

23. Tokayer J, Jia Y, Dhalla A, Huang D. Blood flow velocity quantification using split-spectrum amplitude-decorrelation angiography with optic coherence tomography. Biomed Opt Express. 2013 Oct; 4(10): 1909-24.

24. Jia Y, Bailey S, Wilson D, et al. Quantitative optical coherence tomography angiography of choroidal neovascularization in age-related macular degeneration. Ophthalmology. 2014;121:1435-44.

OCT Angiography Examination of Choroidal Neovascular Membrane in Other Disorders

Maddalena Quaranta-El Maftouhi, Adil El Maftouhi

A new insight in the comprehension and imaging interpretation of several neovascular diseases is now possible, all thanks to OCT angiography.

The aim of this chapter is to give an overview of the use of OCT angiography in some of the more frequent neovascular pathologies of the posterior pole.

TYPE 1 CNV IN CHRONIC CENTRAL SEROUS CHORIORETINOPATHY

First of all, we studied the OCT angiographic appearance of chronic central serous chorioretinopathy (CSC), in which type 1

neovascularization (CNV) has been recently described. Despite the use of a multimodal imaging procedure, it is hard to affirm the presence of CNV and to differentiate which case presents CNV and which is secondarily complicated with a typical polypoidal choroidal vasculopathy (PCV) (Figs 9.1A to D). Using standard OCT examination, we found that chronic CSC can present with 2 different patterns according to the appearance of the RPE complex. Patients could present either with a flat profile of the RPE, or with a slightly elevated and undulating RPE complex. On OCT angiography, all patients with this second RPE complex pattern appeared to be vascularized (Figs 9.2A and B) even when ICG angiography failed to detect any clear sign of

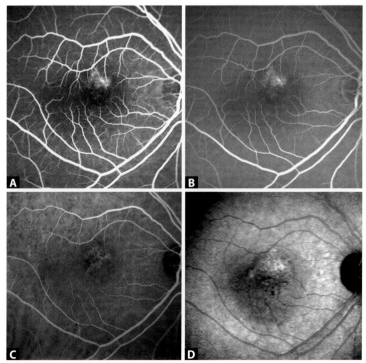

Figs 9.1A to D: (A and B) Fluorescein angiography of the right eye of a 57 years old patient who had been followed for chronic CSC during 6 years. A hyper fluorescent supero-foveal lesion is visible from the early phase angiography, leaving place to a late phase leakage from undetermined source. (C and D) Early and late phases ICG angiography depicting a hyper-fluorescent choroidal vascular network, transforming in a hyperfluorescent late plaque.

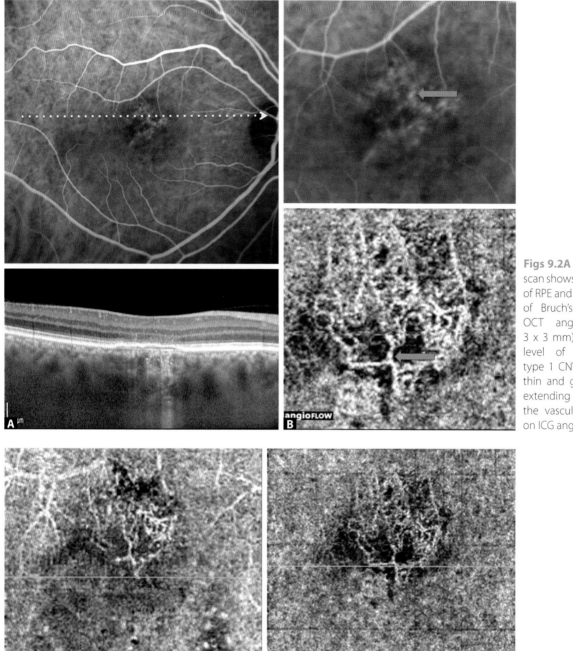

Figs 9.2A and B: (A) OCT B scan shows a slight elevation of RPE and a mild thickening of Bruch's membrane. (B) OCT angiography (Cube 3 x 3 mm) visualizes at the level of undulated RPE, type 1 CNV. CNV appear as thin and granular channels extending largely beyond the vascular network seen on ICG angiography.

Figs 9.3A and B: OCT angiography (Cube 3 x 3 mm) (A) At baseline CNV of CSC present a bullous serous detachment. (B) 3 months after photodynamic therapy with Visudyne, the neovascular network is still perfused, but is no longer exudative.

choroidal neovascularization. New vessels were located between the elevated RPE and the Bruch's membrane (type 1 CNV). The neovascular network was wheel –rays in shape, and presented some dilatations along with the major trunks, but not typical signs of polypoidal dilatations (Figs 9.3A and B).

OCT angiography contributes to clearly give the diagnosis of type 1 CNV secondary to chronic CSC, and allowed to find out that there is a correlation between the slightly elevated and undulated RPE profile on OCT scans and choroidal neovascularization.

POLYPOIDAL CHOROIDAL VASCULOPATHY (PCV)

In polypoidal choroidal vasculopathy (PCV), ICG angiography is pathognomonic. One or multiple early hyperfluorescent spots peripheral or above an interconnecting neovascular network represent the essential clues for diagnosis.

On OCT scans, the polypoidal dilations are dome-shaped elevations of the RPE over an abnormally visible Bruch's membrane. Round, optically empty dots are frequently visible inside the RPE detachment and correspond to the polyp itself. The interconnecting neovascular network appears as an undulated and slightly elevated RPE profile (Figs 9.4A to C).

On OCT angiography (Figs 9.5A and B), both polyps and interconnecting neovascular network are visible under the RPE. The shape of the whole polypoidal complex is shoestring in shape and this aspect is typical of polypoidal lesions. Along with the interconnecting neovascular vessels, some dilatations (polyps) can be seen. However, polyps and neovascular network are not on the same plane and so, their visualization needs the analysis of two or more sequential slabs, the thickness of which have to be adapted to the size of polyps (Fig. 9.6).

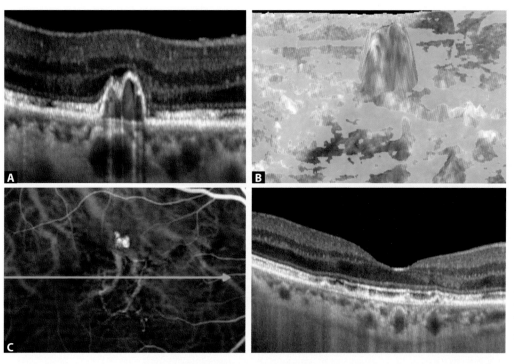

Figs 9.4A to C: (A and B) OCT scan and elevation topography of a polypoidal structure with its typical dome-shape, abrupt elevation of the RPE. (C) The interconnecting neovascular network appears as a slightly elevated and undulated RPE detachment.

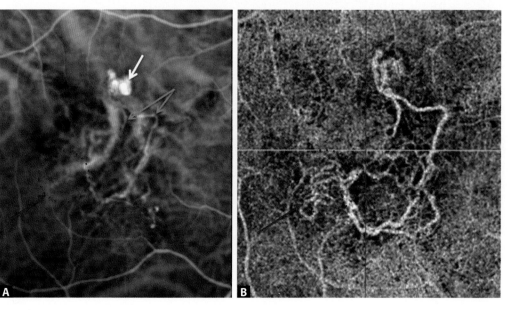

Figs 9.5A and B: (A) On ICG angiography, only the polypoidal lesion (white arrow) and the major vessels of the interconnecting neovascular network (blue arrows) are visible on the early phase frame. B) On OCT angiography, the whole neovascular network can be visualized beneath the RPE. It brings additional information about the extent of the neovascular interconnecting network (red arrow) as compared to ICG angiography.

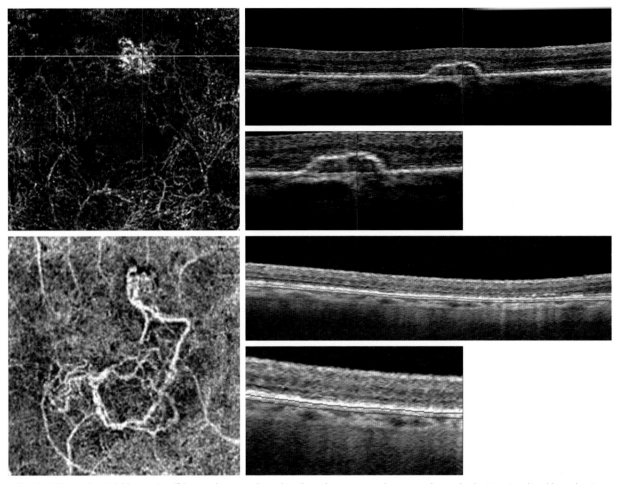

Fig. 9.6: The polypoidal lesion itself, located on another plan than the neovascular network, can be better visualized by selecting appropriate slabs.

CNV IN PATHOLOGIC MYOPIA

Choroidal neovascularization of pathologic myopia is usually small in size and presents a mild late leakage on fluorescein angiography. Despite the fact that myopic CNV are classic and located beneath the RPE, their precise structure is difficult to see on conventional FA. The high sensitivity and specificity of OCT angiography allows visualizing very small CNVs in detail. Major vessels contrast on a hypoperfused zone. It is not yet established if the dark zone encircling and underlying new vessels is due to exudative material or to hypoperfusion. The peripheral fringe of CNV, made of more thin, immature and leaking vessels, seems to present a hazy blood flow which is probably due to an optic attenuation of blood flow signal due to exudation overlying CNV (Figs 9.7A and B)

ANGIOID STREAKS AND CHOROIDAL NEOVASCULARIZATION

Angiod streaks (AS) are breaks of the Bruch's membrane due to a pathologic calcification of elastic tissues. On ICG angiography, we described their late hyperfluorescence scattered with tiny pinpoints. Type 2 CNV can complicate AS and diagnosis is normally based on FA or, only in some more difficult cases, on ICG angiography (Figs 9.8 and 9.9).

On OCT angiography, we could individualize not only type 2 CNV (hyper reflective network localized above the RPE complex), but also type 1 CNV (perfused CNV localized between RPE and Bruch's membrane). Type 1 CNV could be just beside the classic component, but also at distance along the bed of the AS (Figs 9.10A and B).

For the first time, OCT angiography allowed to clarify the neovascular nature of some ICG hyperfluorescences and to diagnose perfused type 1 CNV in AS (Figs 9.11A and B).

The good response of anti-VEGF therapy is very evident in OCT angiography by the lack of decorrelation (Fig. 9.12)

CNV IN MULTIFOCAL CHOROIDITIS

In multifocal choroiditis (MC), classic CNV penetrate under the neurosensory retina through a post-inflammatory discontinuation of Bruch's membrane and RPE (Figs 9.13A and B)

On OCT angiography, CNV are not different from classic CNV of AMD showing a typical sea fan or wheel-rays shape, but type 1 CNV are always absent (Figs 9.14A and B). Anti-VEGF treatment usually obtains a regression of the subretinal neovascular component, but the CNV at the penetration site persists perfused. This persistence can be the reason for further recurrences (Figs 9.15A and B).

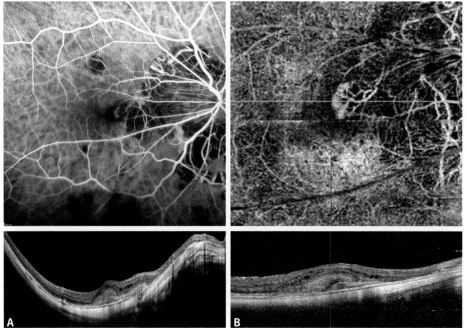

Figs 9.7A and B: A) Fluorescein angiography of classic CNV of pathologic myopia. The small size of CNV does not allow the visualization of the neovascular details due to leakage. (B) On OCT angiography (Cube 3 x 3 mm), thanks to high sensitivity in flow detection, the neovascularization appears constituted of two parts: Hyperreflective larger vessels, contrasting on a hyporeflective background, and a hyperreflective and hazy peripheral fringe. This hazy aspect seems to be correlated with the presence of a diffuse edema.

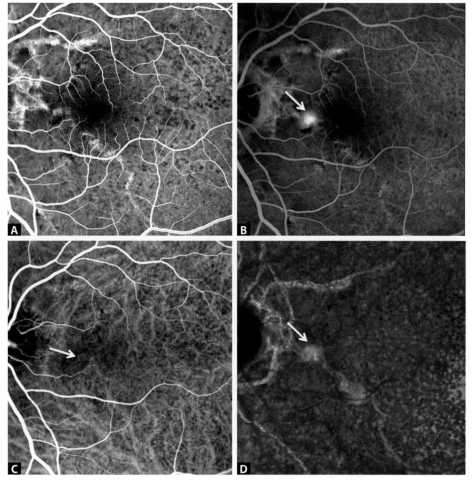

Figs 9.8A to D: (A and B) Fluorescein angiography of classic, late leaking CNV (white arrow) along the bed of the streak. (C and D) ICG angiography barely shows CNV in the early phase frame (white arrow), while the fluffy fluorescence on the late frame allows to differentiating CNV from the hyperfluorescent AS. A second zone of late hyperfluorescence (red arrow) is visualized.

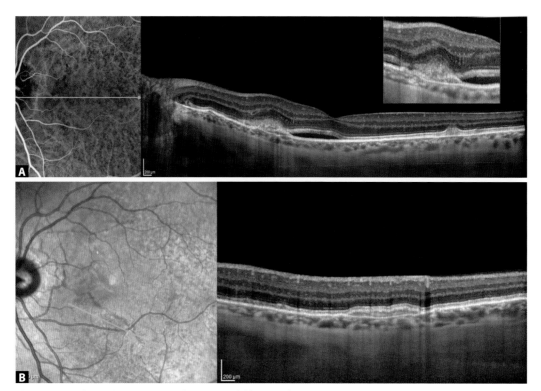

Figs 9.9A and B: (A) OCT B scan depicts a mild hyperreflective subretinal material corresponding to recent classic CNV associated to a small RPE detachment (red arrow). (B) OCT B scan passing on the ICG hyper fluorescent zone visualized along the AS. RPE is elevated by a mildly reflective material.

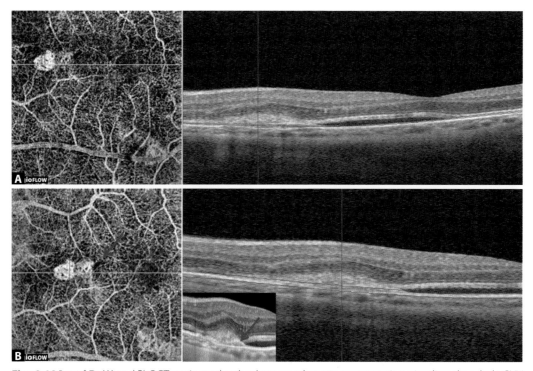

Figs 9.10A and B: (A) and B) OCT angiography, thanks to an adequate segmentation, visualizes the whole CNV and allows to disclosing the presence of an occult component at the level of the small RPE detachment (red arrow).

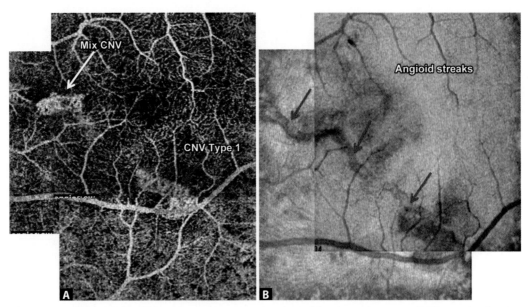

Figs 9.11A and B: (A) On OCT angiographic composite, the mildly elevated zone on OCT scan, localized at distance from CNV appears to be perfused (red arrow). This type 1 CNV is not yet exudative. (B) *En face* OCT composite enable the visualization of AS.

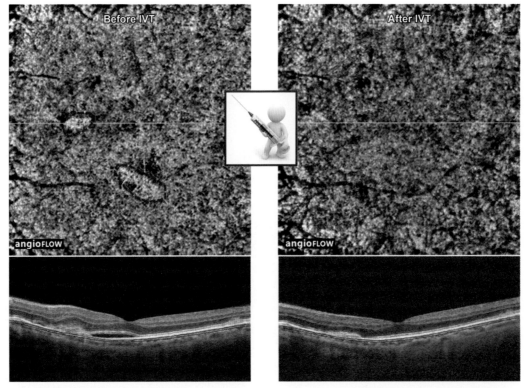

Fig. 9.12: On OCT angiography, occult as well as classic CNVs are no longer perfused one month after anti-VEGF treatment.

PSEUDOVITELLIFORM RETICULAR DYSTROPHY AND CNV

In reticular dystrophy, and in particular in the pseudovitelliform form, the differential diagnosis between late FA staining of material and late leakage from CNV can be a challenge especially in the very early stages of the neovascular complication (Figs 9.16A and B).

The high sensitivity and specificity of OCT angiography allows recognizing vascularized and perfused CNV even in presence of pseudovitelliform material. The presence of a perfused CNV can be detected even before intraretinal exudation and can though be fundamental for early diagnosis and proper management (Figs 9.17A and B).

OCT angiography may provide some information about peculiar details of CNV complicating retinal diseases, which can not be imaged with other techniques. In our experience, OCT angiography is the new fundamental tool for early and proper diagnosis and management of choroidal neovascularization.

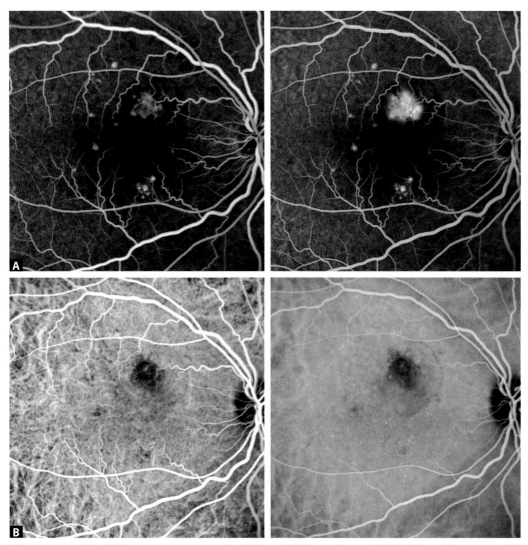

Figs 9.13A and B: (A) Fluorescein angiography of classic CNV secondary to MC. Early hyperfluorescent CNV is encircled by a ring of elevated hypofluorescence. Late leakage masks the details of CNV. Multiple early hyperfluorescent spots due to window defect are the angiographic sign of the past choroiditis. (B) On ICG angiography, the small size of CNV does not allow the visualization of the neovascular details. Choroiditis scars are hypofluorescent.

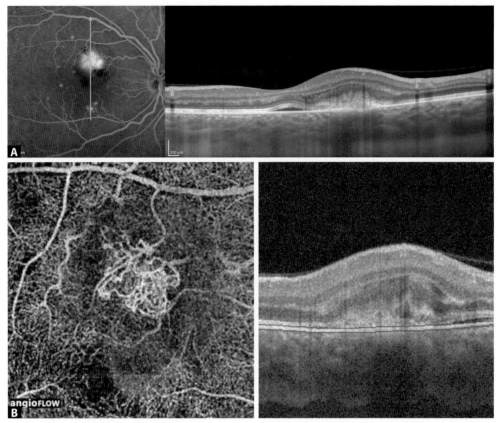

Figs 9.14A and B: (A) OCT scans depicts a mildly reflective subretinal material typical of classic CNV associated with a serous retinal detachment. (B) On OCT angiography (Cube 3 x 3 mm), the sea fan shape neovascularization is perfectly visible as a lace of vessels.

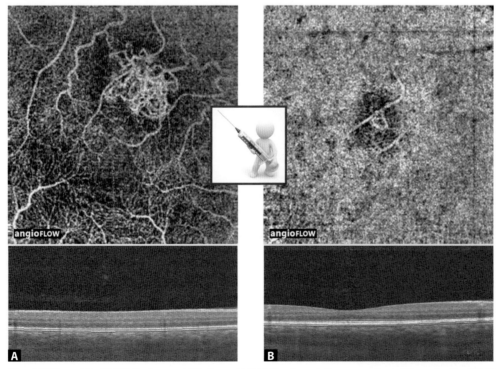

Figs 9.15A and B: (A) CNV before and (B) after anti-VEGF treatment. The regression of the subretinal CNV is complete. Only the vessels at the penetration site (post-inflammatory disruption of Bruch's membrane and RPE) persist perfused.

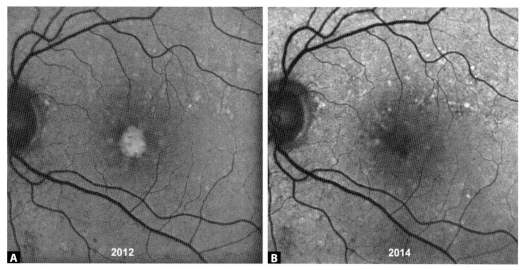

Figs 9.16A and B: Auto fluorescence images of the evolution of a hyper autoreflective material over a period of 2 years. The resorption of the material justifies the disappearance of the foveal hyper autofluorescent spot.

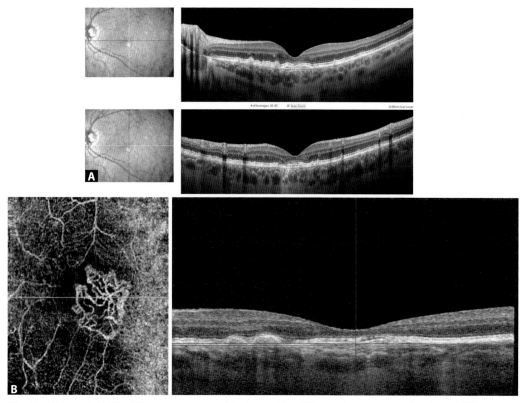

Figs 9.17A and B: (A) On OCT scans some undulations of the RPE complex correspond to drusen. RPE appears altered by some atrophic changes. (B) OCT angiography gives an unexpected diagnosis of perfused type 1 CNV without exudation signs.

BIBLIOGRAPHY

1. Jia Y, Tan O, Tokayer J, Potsaid B, Wang Y, Liu JJ, et al. Split-spectrum amplitude-decorrelation angiography with optical coherence tomography. Opt Express. 2012;20(4):4710-25.

2. Jia Y, Wei E, Wang X, Zhang X, Morrison JC, Parikh M, et al. Optical coherence tomography angiography of optic disc perfusion in glaucoma. Ophthalmology. 2014;121(7):1322-32.doi:10.1016/j.ophtha.2014.01.021. Epub 2014 Mar 12.

3. Spaide RF, Klancnik JM Jr, Cooney MJ. Retinal vascular layers imaged by fluorescein angiography and optical coherence tomography angiography. JAMA Ophthalmol. 20151;133(1):45-50. doi: 10.1001/jamaophthalmol. 2014.3616

4. Jia Y, Bailey ST, Wilson DJ, Tan O, Klein ML, Flaxel CJ, et al. Quantitative optical coherence tomography angiography of choroidal neovascularization in age-related macular degeneration. Ophthalmology. 2014;121(7):1435-44.

5. Lumbroso B, Huang D, Jian Y, Fujimoto JG, Rispoli M. Clinical guide to Angio-OCT. Jaypee. ISBN: 978-93_5152-399-4.

6. Wei E, Jia Y, Tan O, Potsaid B, et al. Parafoveal Retinal Vascular Response to Pattern Visual Stimulation Assessed with OCT Angiography. PLoS ONE. 2012;8(12): e81343. doi:10.1371/journal.pone.0081343.

OCT Angiography Follow-up of Choroidal Neovascularization After Treatment

Bruno Lumbroso, Marco Rispoli

OCT angiography allows to detect CNVs by showing the blood flow without leakage or staining. This noninvasive procedure gives the possibility to perform several examinations in order to follow closely the treatment results. We report OCT angiographic measurement of the CNV response to treatment in two clinical cases.

Software may segment CNVs in several ways. It is possible to study type 1, type 2 and type 3 CNVs.

We applied on two patients an experimental software that shows indirectly the blood flow inside the CNV (average pixel density) and the CNV area, correlated with the intravitreal injections and visual acuity.

These cases confirm Lumbroso and Huang publication and show that re-opening of CNV vessels occurs generally 2 weeks prior to fluid re-accumulation. Larger studies are needed to confirm that CNV flow and area are leading indicators that precede fluid accumulation and visual decline. If confirmed, then OCT angiography might be useful in guiding the interval between injections so that fluid re-accumulation does not occur. It is also intriguing whether more frequent injections that do not allow the re-opening of CNV channels might affect earlier and more permanent CNV regression (Figs 10.1 to 10.7).

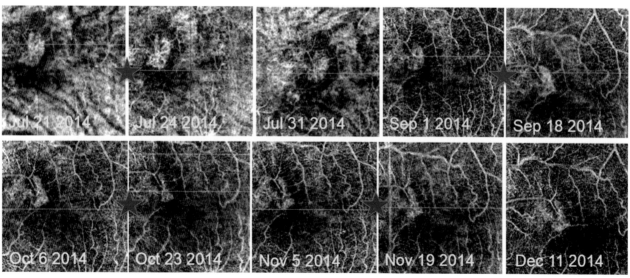

Fig. 10.1: Angioflow sequence of CNV treated with Aflibercept injections. We can clearly see the CNV network. Red star indicates the Aflibercept injection.

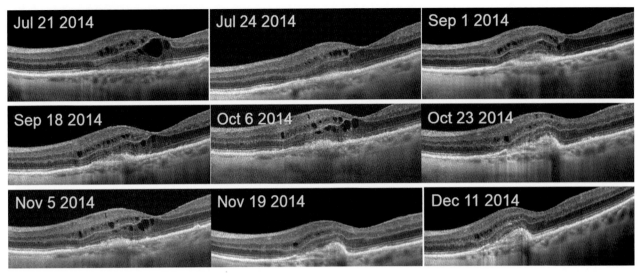

Fig. 10.2: B-scan structural sequence correlated to the angioflow images. *Note* the progressive CME resorption.

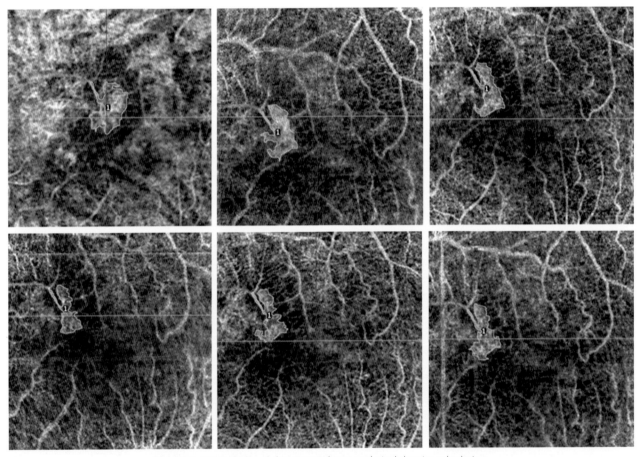

Fig. 10.3: CNV area hand drawing and area and pixel density calculation.

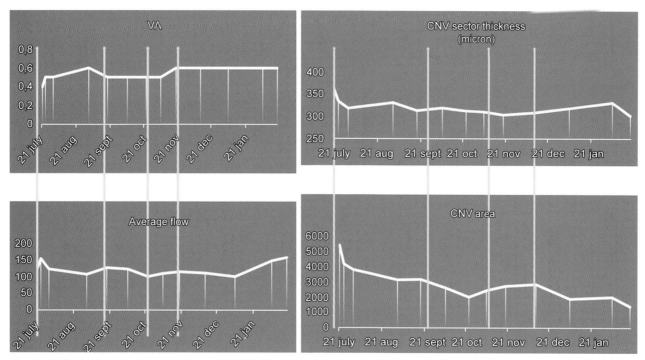

Fig. 10.4: Graph correlating visual acuity, indirect CNV flow, macula thickness and CNV area during the follow up. Yellow arrows indicate intravitreal injections.

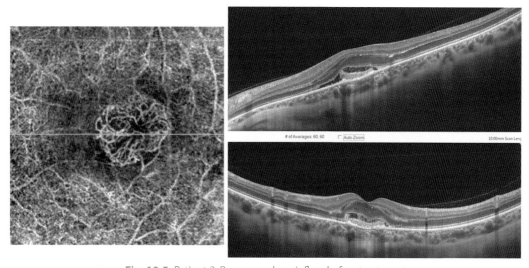

Fig. 10.5: Patient 2: B-scans and angioflow before treatment.

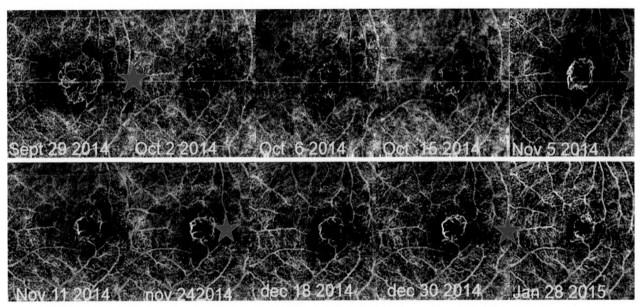

Fig. 10.6: Angioflow sequence of CNV treated with Aflibercept. We can clearly see the CNV network. Red stars indicate Ranibizumab injection.

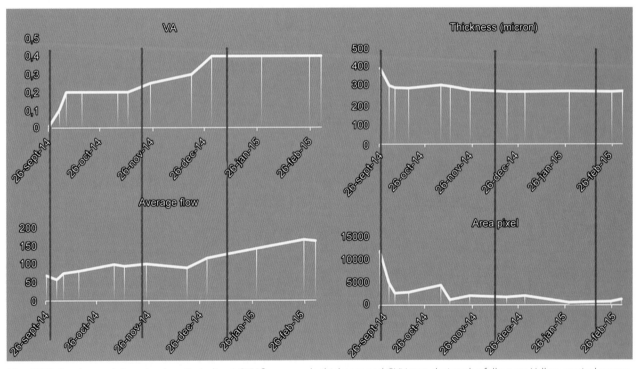

Fig. 10.7: Graph correlating visual acuity, indirect CNV flow, macula thickness and CNV area during the follow up. Yellow vertical arrows indicate the intravitreal injections.

Non-neovascular Age-related Macular Degeneration

*Talisa de Carlo, Eric Moult, WooJhon Choi,
Nadia K Waheed, Jay S Duker, James G Fujimoto*

INTRODUCTION

Non-neovascular or dry age-related macular degeneration (AMD) is characterized by drusen and pigmentary alterations in the early stages and photoreceptor and RPE loss (geographic atrophy, GA) in the late stages of the disease. Blood flow alterations in non-neovascular AMD can occur in two distinct ways: when there is progression to the neovascular form of AMD, and when the choroidal circulation is altered, either as a primary cause or a secondary event. For example, increased drusen extent has been associated with decreased foveolar choroidal blood flow, which has been hypothesized to predict disease progression.[1]

OCT angiography (OCTA) is capable of visualizing the choriocapillaris blood flow, and therefore, may have use in the evaluation of non-neovascular AMD. Areas of choriocapillaris alteration are easily visualized using an en face OCTA image plane immediately below Bruch's membrane. Since OCTA visualizes blood flow using motion contrast, choriocapillaris alterations on OCTA may represent either choriocapillaris atrophy (no flow) or impaired blood flow. If the blood flow velocity is below the sensitivity threshold of the OCTA acquisition, which is determined by the interscan time between repeat OCT B-scans, vasculature will not be visible by OCTA and therefore, might be mistaken as atrophy. To avoid this misinterpretation, the interscan time of the OCTA acquisition can be increased, which increases the sensitivity of OCTA (i.e. lowers the slowest detectable flow), and slower flows can be detected. However, increasing the interscan time also increases the susceptibility of OCTA to parasitic eye motion and noise. For these reasons, the interscan time is an important parameter in OCTA imaging. The time between repeat OCT B-scans is ~1.5 ms for the swept source OCT (SS-OCT) prototype from the Massachusetts Institute of Technology (Department of Electrical Engineering and Computer Science, Cambridge, MA) and ~5 ms for the spectral domain OCT (SD-OCT) device from Optovue Inc. (Fremont, CA).

EARLY STAGES

OCTA imaging of the choriocapillaris in normal eyes shows a dense homogeneous network, which has a lobular pattern peripheral in the retina and has a fine pattern in the macula, in which it is difficult to discern individual capillaries. These patterns are observed using both SD-OCT, centered at an 840 nm wavelength, and SS-OCT, centered at a 1,050 nm wavelength (Fig. 11.1). The SS-OCT provides deeper choroidal penetration at this wavelength. Non-neovascular AMD eyes appear to have a generalized decrease in choriocapillaris density and, in some cases, focal areas of choriocapillaris loss. In mild dry AMD eyes featuring only a few hard and soft drusen, OCTA using an SS-OCT system demonstrates decreased choriocapillaris density as evidenced by dark patches in the choriocapillaris, allowing larger vessels to be seen (Fig. 11.2, SS-OCT at 1,050 nm). These changes become more marked in more severe cases. In non-neovascular AMD eyes, where OCT B-scans exhibit disruption of the outer retinal layers, SS-OCTA shows a dramatic decrease in choriocapillaris density (Fig. 11.3, SS-OCT at 1,050 nm). In these cases, it is sometimes-possible to see larger choroidal vessels that have been displaced into the space previously occupied by the choriocapillaris (Fig. 11.3 C and D).

Since the en face OCTA images (angiograms) are co-registered with their corresponding structural OCT B-scans, the OCT B-scans can be scrolled through in the same manner as a cube scan. Therefore, corresponding OCT B-scans can be viewed at a specific cross-section of the OCT angiogram. In this fashion, it can be shown that some drusen seen on the corresponding OCT b-scans are associated with underlying areas of choriocapillaris alteration. However, some drusen contain dense material that causes shadowing on the choriocapillaris, especially using a SD-OCT device due to its lower wavelength of 840 nm. This can show up as a signal attenuation artifact with decreased signal below the druse on the corresponding OCT B-scans, and also as a loss

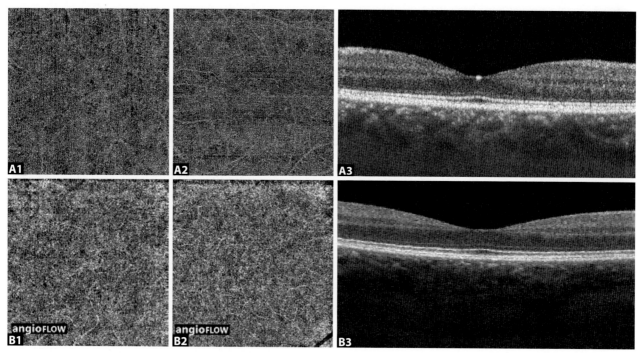

Fig. 11.1A to C: (A) OCTA images obtained using a prototype swept source OCT system at 1050 nm wavelength (Department of Electrical Engineering and Computer Science, Massachusetts Institute of Technology, Cambridge, MA) of the normal left eye of a 40-year-old Caucasian woman. Choriocapillaris is generally dense and homogeneous. 3 mm x 3 mm (A1) and 6 mm x 6 mm (A2) en face OCTAs, and a 3 mm OCT B-scan (A3). (B) Images obtained using the Angiovue optical coherence tomography angiography (OCTA) software of the RTVue XR Avanti spectral domain OCT system at 840 nm wavelength (Optovue, Inc., Fremont, CA) of the normal right eye of a 28-year-old Caucasian woman. 3 mm x 3 mm (B1) and 6 mm x 6 mm (B2) en face OCTAs, and a 3 mm OCT b-scan (B3). The swept source OCT has deeper choroidal penetration but the spectral domain OCT has better axial resolution.

of signal on the OCTA that mimics choriocapillaris loss (Figs 11.4 and 11.5, SD-OCT at 840 nm). The OCTA choriocapillaris "loss" below drusen should be interpreted with caution because this may be an attenuation artifact where OCTA does not show choriocapillaris flow even though it may be present. Figure 13.6 shows two eyes with non-neovascular AMD imaged on the same day with a SD-OCT and SS-OCT device. The OCTA from the SD-OCT demonstrated attenuation artifact not seen on the SS-OCT OCTA images.

LATE STAGES

In patients with geographic atrophy (GA), OCTA with a SS-OCT device shows a near total atrophy of choriocapillaris underneath the regions of GA. In some cases, the choriocapillaris alterations may extend beyond the GA margins or between discrete areas of GA (Fig. 11.7, SS-OCT at 1050 nm). In other cases, the choriocapillaris alterations are subtler, continuing slightly past the GA boundaries (Figs 11.8 and 11.9, SS-OCT at 1,050 nm). Finally, other cases show that the borders of the GA and the choriocapillaris loss are almost exactly the same (Figs 11.10 and 11.11, SS-OCT at 1,050 nm). OCTA of the choriocapillaris in cases of GA also typically displays larger choroidal vessels displaced into the areas of decreased choriocapillaris. Therefore these vessels can be seen on en face OCTA at the depth level of the choriocapillaris (Figs 11.7 to 11.11, SS-OCT at 1,050 nm; Figs 11.12 and 11.13, SD-OCT 840 nm). Because SD-OCT has less

image penetration below the RPE and drusen, it can be difficult to visualize choriocapillaris changes which are in regions peripheral to GA, although in the region of GA more obvious changes can be seen, such as larger choroidal vessels displaced upwards or a sparser, more heterogeneous-appearing choriocapillaris (Figs 11.12 and 11.13, SD-OCT 840 nm).

There has been debate about whether the primary site of pathogenesis of GA is the choriocapillaris or the RPE. Recently it has been suggested that choriocapillaris loss precedes the RPE atrophy.[2] Using SS-OCTA and varying the interscan time in order to vary the flow detection sensitivity, it can be shown that choriocapillaris alterations within the borders of GA tend to be primarily atrophic, while choriocapillaris alterations beyond the borders typically correspond to impaired flow. The OCTA findings that choriocapillaris alterations appear to be at least the size of the GA, and often greater, may support the hypothesis that choriocapillaris loss may precede RPE changes.

In summary, OCTA can be used to visualize alterations in the choriocapillaris, which are present at all stages of disease. OCTA using a SS-OCT device has increased choroidal penetration and thus shows less signal attenuation artifact and provides enhanced OCTA resolution when compared to OCTA using an SD-OCT device. OCTA assessment of the choriocapillaris may be of diagnostic use in the future for detecting and monitoring non-neovascular AMD changes and understanding disease progression.

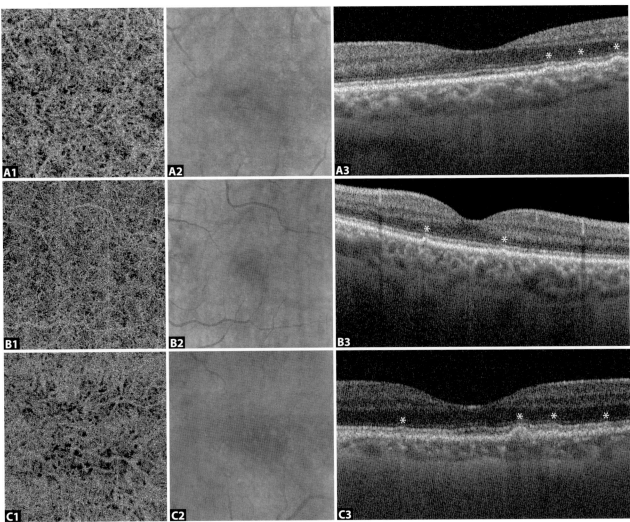

Fig. 11.2: OCTA images obtained using a prototype swept source OCT system at 1050 nm wavelength (Department of Electrical Engineering and Computer Science, Massachusetts Institute of Technology, Cambridge, MA). (A and B) 3 mm x 3 mm (A) and 6 mm x 6 mm (B) OCTA images of the left eye of a 75-year-old Caucasian man with non-neovascular age-related macular degeneration (AMD). (A1, B1) OCT angiogram demonstrating diffusely decreased choriocapillaris density. (A2, B2) En-face intensity OCT of the retinal pigment epithelium (RPE) showing hypo-pigmented lesions representing drusen. (A3, B3) OCT B-scan showing deposits under the RPE signifying drusen (white *). (C) 3 mm x 3 mm images of the right eye of a 73-year-old Caucasian man with non-neovascular AMD. (C1) OCTA demonstrating diffusely decreased choriocapillaris density. (C2) En-face intensity OCT of the retinal pigment epithelium (RPE) showing hypo-pigmented lesions representing drusen (C3) OCT B-scan showing deposits under the RPE signifying drusen (white *).

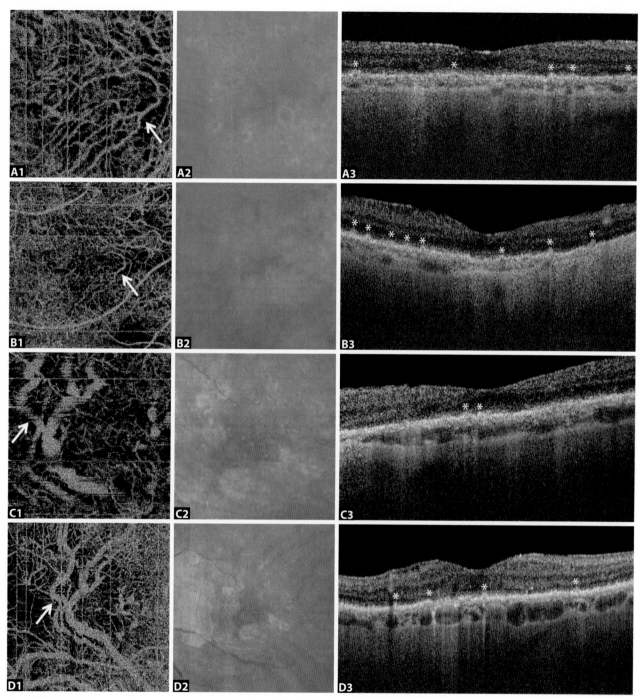

Fig. 11.3: OCTA images obtained using a prototype swept source OCT system at 1050 nm wavelength (Department of Electrical Engineering and Computer Science, Massachusetts Institute of Technology, Cambridge, MA). (A to D) 3 mm x 3 mm (A) and 6 mm x 6 mm (B) OCTA images of the right eye and 3 mm x 3 mm (C) and 6 mm x 6 mm (D) images of the left eye of an 87-year-old Caucasian woman with non-neovascular age-related macular degeneration (AMD). (A1, B1, C1, D1) OCTA exhibiting diffuse severely decreased choriocapillaris density. Larger choroidal vessels have been displaced into the choriocapillaris space, and therefore, can be seen in these en face images (white arrows). (A2, B2, C2, D2) En-face intensity OCT of the retinal pigment epithelium (RPE) showing hypo-pigmented lesions representing drusen (A3, B3, C3, D3) OCT B-scans showing deposits under the RPE signifying drusen (white *). The three hyper-reflective bands corresponding to the ellipsoid layer, RPE, and Bruch's membrane are difficult to discern.

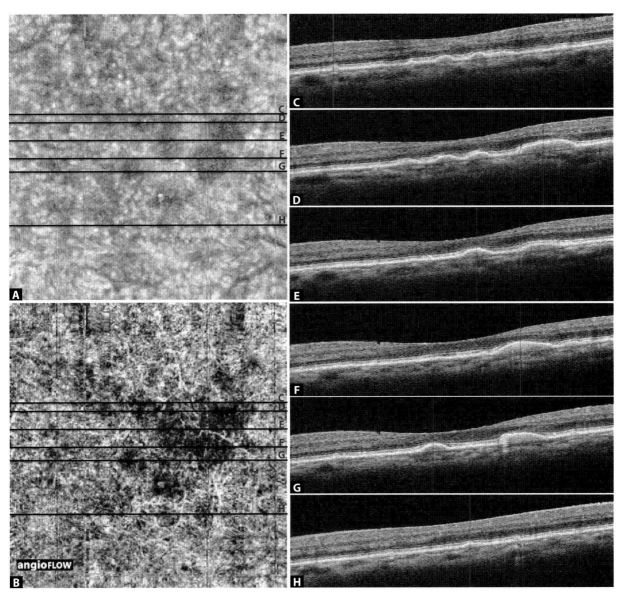

Figs 11.4A to H: Images obtained using the angiovue optical coherence tomography angiography (OCTA) software of the RTVue XR Avanti spectral domain OCT system at 840 nm wavelength (Optovue, Inc., Fremont, CA). 3 mm x 3 mm OCT and OCTA of the left eye of an 81-year-old Asian woman with non-neovascular age-related macular degeneration (AMD). En-face intensity OCT of the choriocapillaris (A) and OCTA of the choriocapillaris (B) showing areas of attenuated signal. The images are marked with the cross-sectional location of the corresponding X-axis OCT B-scans (C to H). The drusen shown on the OCT B-scans are associated with areas of decreased signal in the choriocapillaris, which could be mistaken for flow impairment. (H) demonstrates decreased signal in the choriocapillaris under the druse but to a much lesser degree. The hard druse in (C) is not directly associated with underlying choriocapillaris alterations.

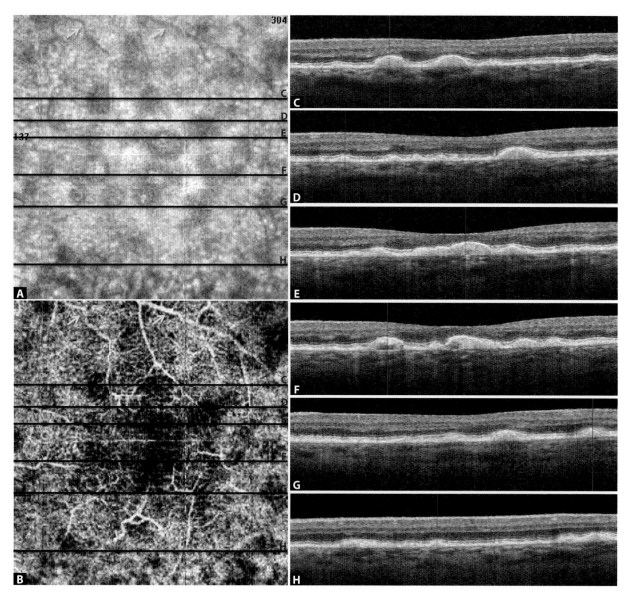

Figs 11.5A to H: Images obtained using the Angiovue optical coherence tomography angiography (OCTA) software of the RTVue XR Avanti spectral domain OCT instrument at 840 nm wavelength (Optovue, Inc., Fremont, CA). 3 mm x 3 mm images of the left eye of a 69-year-old Caucasian woman with non-neovascular age-related macular degeneration (AMD). En-face intensity OCT of the choriocapillaris (B) and OCTA of the choriocapillaris (C) showing areas of attenuated signal and angiographic shadowing from the retinal vasculature (yellow arrows). The images are marked with the cross-sectional location of the corresponding X-axis OCT B-scans (C-H). The drusen shown on the OCT B-scans are associated with areas of decreased signal in the choriocapillaris, which could be mistaken for flow impairment. The drusen in (D) and (H) are not directly associated with underlying choriocapillaris alterations.

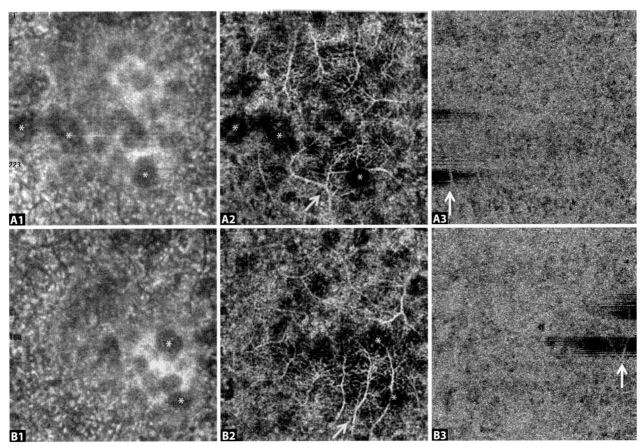

Figs 11.6A and B: OCTA images of the right (A) and left (B) eyes of a 74-year-old Caucasian man with non-neovascular age-related macular degeneration (AMD). (A1-A2, B1-B2) Images obtained using the Angiovue optical coherence tomography angiography (OCTA) software of the RTVue XR Avanti spectral domain OCT system at 840 nm wavelength (Optovue, Inc., Fremont, CA). *En face* intensity OCT of the choriocapillaris (A1, B1) and OCTA of the choriocapillaris (A2, B2) showing areas of attenuated signal (white *) and angiographic shadowing from the retinal vasculature (yellow arrows). (A3, B3) OCTA images obtained using a prototype swept source OCT system at 1050 nm wavelength (Department of Electrical Engineering and Computer Science, Massachusetts Institute of Technology, Cambridge, MA) does not demonstrate attenuation artifact. However, segmentation error artifacts are seen (white arrows).

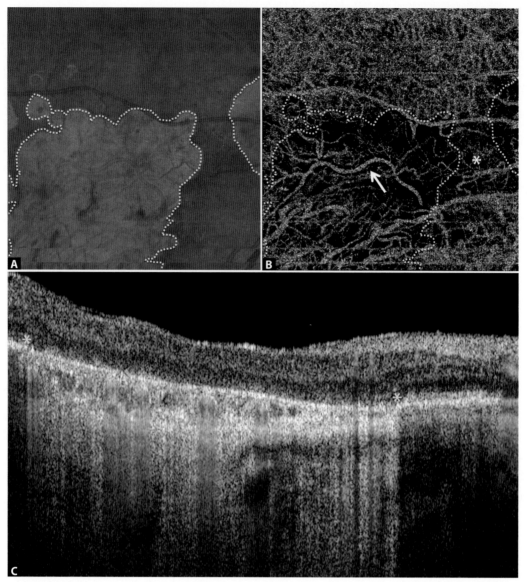

Figs 11.7A to C: OCTA images obtained using a prototype swept source OCT system (Department of Electrical Engineering and Computer Science, Massachusetts Institute of Technology, Cambridge, MA). 6 mm x 6 mm images of an 82-year old Caucasian woman with geographic atrophy (GA) due to non-neovascular age-related macular degeneration (AMD) (A) En-face intensity OCT at the level of the RPE demonstrating two discrete areas of GA. The areas of GA are circumscribed in yellow, which are overlaid over the image in B. (B) OCTA at the level of the choriocapillaris demonstrating flow impairment in a similar area as the GA. The choriocapillaris alterations extend beyond the GA borders and between the two areas of GA (white *). Larger choroidal vessels have been displaced into the area of choriocapillaris alteration so are seen in this 10 um thick slab (white arrow). C) Corresponding OCT B-scan shows the loss of RPE (between the two yellow *) causing increased intensity below Bruch's membrane which is the characteristic of GA.

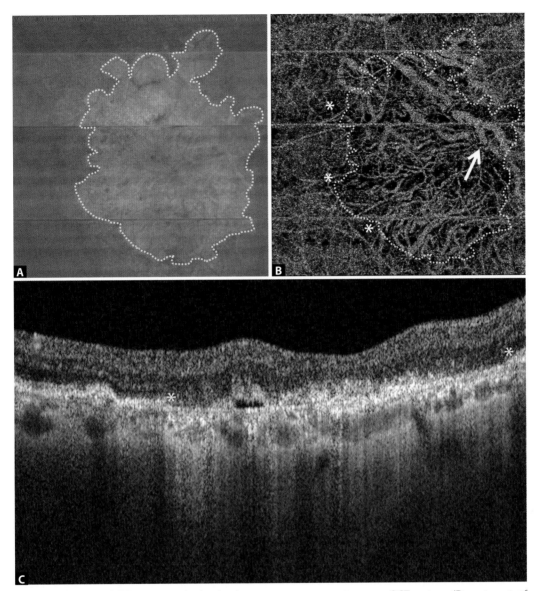

Figs 11.8A to C: OCTA images obtained using a prototype swept source OCT system (Department of Electrical Engineering and Computer Science, Massachusetts Institute of Technology, Cambridge, MA). 6 mm x 6 mm images of a 76-year-old Caucasian man with geographic atrophy (GA) due to non-neovascular age-related macular degeneration (AMD) (A) En-face intensity OCT at the level of the RPE demonstrating GA. The area of GA is circumscribed in yellow, which is overlaid over the image in B. (B) OCT angiogram at the level of the choriocapillaris demonstrating flow impairment in a similar area as the GA. The choriocapillaris changes extend slightly beyond the GA borders (white *). Larger choroidal vessels have been displaced into the area of choriocapillaris alteration so they are seen in this 10 um thick slab (white arrow). C) Corresponding OCT B-scan shows the loss of RPE (between the two yellow *) causing increased intensity below Bruch's membrane which is the characteristic of GA.

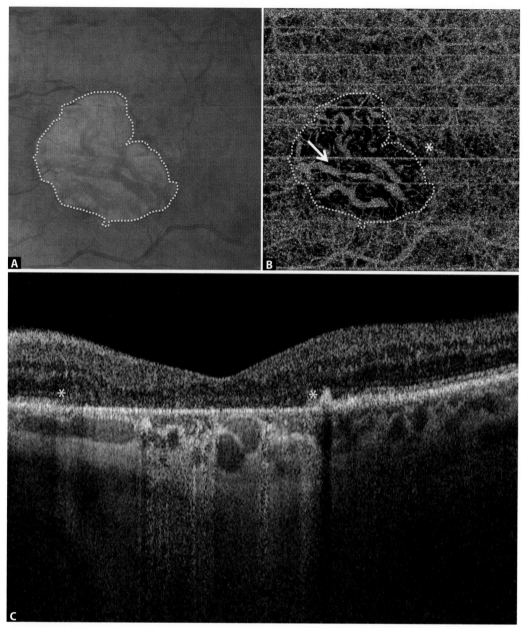

Figs 11.9A to C: OCTA images obtained using a prototype swept source OCT system (Department of Electrical Engineering and Computer Science, Massachusetts Institute of Technology, Cambridge, MA). 6 mm x 6 mm images of a 76-year-old Caucasian man with geographic atrophy (GA) due to non-neovascular age-related macular degeneration (AMD) (A) En-face intensity OCT at the level of the RPE demonstrating GA. The area of GA is circumscribed in yellow, which is overlaid over the image in B. (B) OCT angiogram at the level of the choriocapillaris demonstrating flow impairment in a similar area as the GA. The choriocapillaris changes extend slightly beyond the GA borders (white *). Larger choroidal vessels have been displaced into the choriocapillaris space so they are seen in this 10 um thick slab (white arrow). (C) Corresponding OCT B-scan shows the loss of RPE (between the two yellow *) causing increased intensity below Bruch's membrane which is the characteristic of GA.

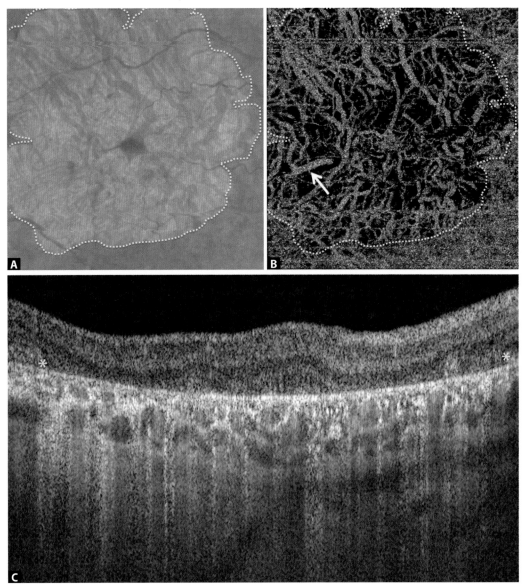

Figs 11.10A to C: OCTA images obtained using a prototype swept source OCT system (Department of Electrical Engineering and Computer Sciences, Massachusetts Institute of Technology, Cambridge, MA). 6 mm x 6 mm images of a 65-year-old Caucasian man with geographic atrophy (GA) due to non-neovascular age-related macular degeneration (AMD) (A) En-face intensity OCT at the level of the RPE demonstrating GA. The area of GA is circumscribed in yellow, which is overlaid over the image in B. (B) OCTA at the level of the choriocapillaris demonstrating flow impairment in almost exactly the same area as the GA. Larger choroidal vessels have been displaced into the choriocapillaris space so they are seen in this 10 um thick slab (white arrow). (C) Corresponding OCT B-scan shows the loss of RPE (between the two yellow *) causing increased intensity below Bruch's membrane which is the characteristic of GA.

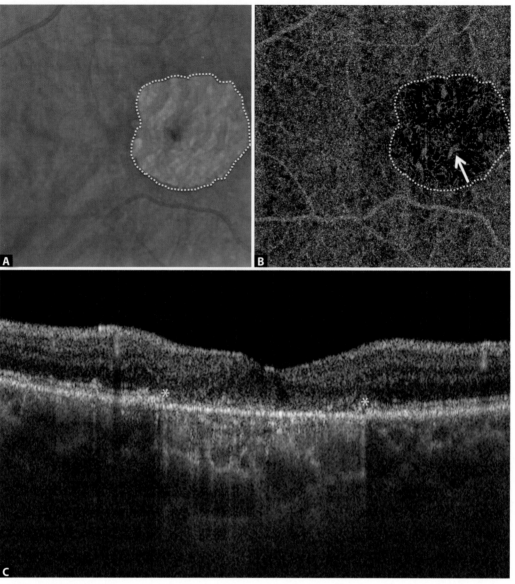

Figs 11.11A to C: OCTA images obtained using a prototype swept source OCT system (Department of Electrical Engineering and Computer Science, Massachusetts Institute of Technology, Cambridge, MA). 6 mm x 6 mm images of a 70-year-old Caucasian man with geographic atrophy (GA) due to non-neovascular age-related macular degeneration (AMD) (A) En-face intensity OCT at the level of the RPE demonstrating GA. The area of GA is circumscribed in yellow, which is overlaid over the image in B. (B) OCT angiogram at the level of the choriocapillaris demonstrating flow impairment in almost exactly the same area as the GA. Larger choroidal vessels have been displaced into the choriocapillaris space so are seen in this 10 um thick slice (white arrow). C) Corresponding OCT B-scan shows the loss of RPE (between the two yellow *) causing increased intensity below Bruch's membrane which is characteristic of GA.

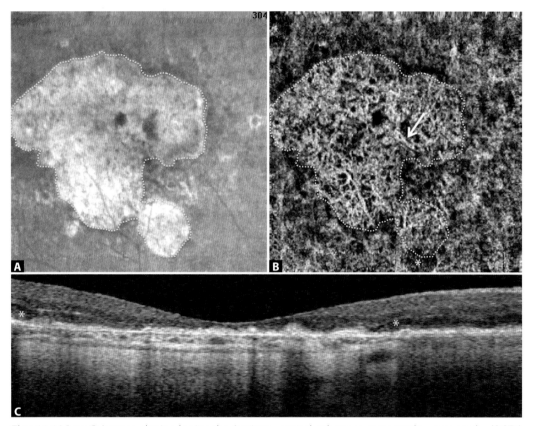

Figs 11.12A to C: Images obtained using the Angiovue optical coherence tomography angiography (OCTA) software of the RTVue XR Avanti spectral domain OCT system at 840 nm wavelength (Optovue, Inc., Fremont, CA). 3 mm x 3 mm images of an 85-year-old Caucasian woman with geographic atrophy (GA) due to non-neovascular age-related macular degeneration (AMD) (A) En-face intensity OCT at the level of the RPE demonstrating GA. The area of GA is circumscribed in yellow, which is overlaid over the image in B. (B) OCT angiogram at the level of the choriocapillaris demonstrating flow impairment in a similar area as the GA. The resolution is greatly reduced compared with the SS-OCT images, therefore, the choriocapillaris changes are difficult to appreciate. The choriocapillaris appears less homogeneous inside the GA borders in some places and extending slightly beyond the GA borders in other locations (white *). Larger choroidal vessels have been displaced into the choriocapillaris space so are seen in this 10 um thick slice (white arrow). (C) Corresponding OCT B-scan shows the loss of RPE (between the two yellow *) causing increased intensity below Bruch's membrane which is the characteristic of GA.

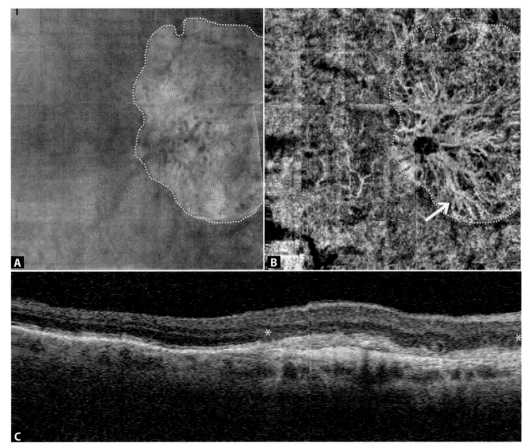

Figs 11.13A to C: . Images obtained using the Angiovue optical coherence tomography angiography (OCTA) software of the RTVue XR Avanti spectral domain OCT system at 840 nm wavelength (Optovue, Inc., Fremont, CA). 6 mm x 6 mm images of an 87-year-old Caucasian woman with geographic atrophy (GA) due to non-neovascular age-related macular degeneration (AMD) (A) En-face intensity OCT at the level of the RPE demonstrating GA. The area of GA is circumscribed in yellow, which is overlaid over the image in B. (B) OCT angiogram at the level of the choriocapillaris demonstrating flow impairment in a similar area as the GA. The resolution is greatly reduced compared with the SD-OCT 3 mm x 3 mm images and the SS-OCT images, therefore, the choriocapillaris changes are difficult to appreciate. The choriocapillaris appears less homogeneous inside the GA borders. Larger choroidal vessels have been displaced into the choriocapillaris space so are seen in this 10 um thick slice (white arrow). (C) Corresponding OCT B-scan shows the loss of RPE (between the two yellow *) causing increased intensity below Bruch's membrane which is characteristic of GA.

REFERENCES

1. Bressler NM, Bressler SB. Neovascular (Exudative or "Wet") Age-Related Macular Degeneration. In: Ryan SJ, Sadda SR, Hinton DR, (Eds). Retina. London: Elsevier Saunders. 2013. pp. 1183-212.

2. Biesemeier A, Taubitz T, Julien S, Yoeruek E, Schraermayer U. Choriocapillaris breakdown precedes retinal degeneration in age-related macular degeneration. Neurobiology of Aging. 2014;35:2562-73.

OCT Angiography Findings in Central Serous Chorioretinopathy

Marco Bonini Filho, Talisa de Carlo, Eric M Moult,
WooJhon Choi, James G Fujimoto, Jay S Duker, Nadia K Waheed

INTRODUCTION

Central serous chorioretinopathy (CSCR) is a relatively common cause of vision loss that affects predominantly young and middle-aged patients, more commonly men than women.[1] The etiology of this disease remains incompletely understood with systemic associations and a complex pathogenesis that involves diffuse dysfunction of the RPE cells, the choroid, or both, regardless of the primary cause or the initiating event.[1-3] The main risk factors for CSCR are systemic corticosteroid use, type A personality, pregnancy and endogenous Cushing's syndrome.[3] Although several clinical presentations are described, the acute form of CSCR is the most common and is characterized by detachment of the neurosensory retina often with one or more areas of retinal pigment epithelium detachments (RPED).[3] Leakage areas from a disrupted RPE barrier and abnormal egress of fluid into the subretinal space are evident during fluorescein angiography (FA), with most patients having blot or dot-like leaks and the minority having smokestack leaks.[1] Indocyanine-green angiography (ICGA) shows respectively choroidal hyperpermeability and vascular congestion.[2] Symptoms are self-limited and resolve spontaneously in 2–3 months in most cases of acute classic CSCR, but the disease can be recurrent or bilateral in approximately one-third of cases.[4,5] Widespread diffuse RPE pigmentary abnormalities including RPE atrophy, cystic retinal-changes, subretinal fibrinous accumulation, subretinal fibrosis, and secondary choroidal neovascularization (CNV) are known as late complications related to permanent visual loss and are observed in the chronic form of CSCR.[1,6]

Optical coherence tomography (OCT) provides both qualitative (morphology and reflectivity) and quantitative (thickness, mapping and volume) analyses of the macula in real time. On OCT B-scans, increased choroidal thickness is found to be a hallmark of CSCR. Classically, one or more sharply demarcated RPEDs with low internal reflectivity and subretinal fluid accumulation with hyper-reflectivity in the level of outer nuclear layer (ONL) are observed in active CSCR[7] (Table 12.1). In chronic forms, OCT B-scans show additional atrophic and cystic changes in the intraretinal layers. RPEDs with heterogeneous high internal reflectivity are observed in some cases, indicating presence of sub-RPE fibrin accumulation, subretinal fibrosis or CNV[8,9] (Table 12.2). Three-dimensional OCT is an additional useful tool to visualize pathologic features at the RPE and choroid layers in eyes with CSCR. Features such as RPE loss extension and choroidal vessels dilation at variable depths can be visualized by using high-speed, enhanced-depth swept-source OCT (SS-OCT) or enhanced depth imaging on the standard spectral domain OCT systems.[9]

Optical coherence tomography angiography (OCTA) is a non-invasive medical imaging technique that enables distinct, depth resolved, three-dimensional visualization of the choriocapillaris and retinal microvasculature by combining vascular flow visualization using motion contrast (OCT angiograms) and structural (co-registered OCT B-scans) information. Detecting CNV in CSCR eyes using dye-based angiography may be challenging due to the coexistence of some confounding features related to the primary diagnosis of CSCR that may be present even in the absence of CNV, such as RPED, subretinal fluid, cystoid macular edema and diffuse irregular hyperfluorescence. Therefore, OCTA is especially helpful for the definitive diagnosis of CNV in this condition.

Table 12.1: Multimodal imaging features of classic/active CSCR

Imaging technique	Features
Fluorescein angiography (FA)	*Early phases:* Focal leaks at the RPE level; *Late phases:* Pooling of the dye into the serous retinal detachment (SRD).
Indocyanine-green angiography (ICGA)	*Early phase:* Areas of lobular hypoperfusion; *Mid phase:* Multiple patches of hyperfluorescence in the inner choroid; *Late phase:* Visualization of silhouetting of the larger choroidal vessels (venous congestion) and dispersion of the hyperfluorescent patches.
OCT B-scan	*Intraretinal layers:* None or minimal changes in retina thickness, fading of photoreceptor band, elongation of outer segments and narrowing of the outer nuclear layer (ONL) layer in the detached neurosensory retina; *Subretinal fluid:* Optically empty space usually related to hyper-reflective deposits underneath the detached retina; *RPE layer:* Small dome-shaped RPEDs with low internal reflectivity and distinct borders; *Choroid:* Choroidal thickening (commonly greater than 500 μm).
en face OCT	*Subretinal fluid:* Hyporeflective area surrounded with concentric circles of retinal layers. Inside the SRD, small hyper-reflective deposits can be seen; *RPE layer:* Highly hyperreflective layer. Small, circular RPEDs with uniform appearance of the reflective wall. *Choroid layers:* Choriocapillaris presents normal aspect or with hyperreflective spots under the area of subretinal fluid representing disease activity ; hyporeflective, dilated choroidal vessels in inner choroid.

Table 12.2: Multimodal imaging features of chronic CSCR

Imaging technique	Features
Fluorescein angiography (FA)	*Early phase:* Areas of granular hyperfluorescence containing one or multiple subtle leakage of dye; *Late phase:* Intraretinal leakage (intraretinal cysts), hyperfluorescent atrophic changes, significant leakage related to CNV areas.
Indocyanine-green Angiography (ICGA)	*Early phase:* Areas of lobular hypoperfusion; *Midphase:* Multiple patches of hyperfluorescence in the inner choroid; *Late phase:* Blockage vs. staining of subretinal deposits (depends on composition), significant leakage related to CNV areas
OCT B-scan	*Intraretinal layers:* Outer retina thinning with or without cystoid cavities; *Subretinal fluid:* Inconstant SRD; fibrinoid/lipids deposits; *RPE:* Multiple dome-shaped RPEDs with heterogenous internal reflectivity; *Choroid:* Choroidal thickening (commonly greater than 500 μm).
En face OCT	*Subretinal fluid:* Hyporeflective area surrounded by concentric circles of retinal layers. Inside the SRD, small hyper-reflective deposits can be seen; *Cystoid cavities or degenerations* can be present at retinal layers level; *RPE layer:* Highly hyperreflective layer. If CNV is present, PEDs with irregular wall aspect can be observed; *Choroid layers:* Choriocapillaris presents normal aspect or with hyperreflective spots under the area of subretinal fluid representing disease activity; hyporeflective, dilated choroidal vessels in inner choroid.

Most of the following data on OCTA in CSCR was obtained with a spectral domain OCT (SD-OCT; RTVue XR Avanti, Optovue, Inc, Fremont, CA) imaging at 840 nm wavelenght. Two automated segmentation lines referencing the outer retina on the coregistered OCT B-scans were manually fine-tuned to be located at the outer border of the outer plexiform layer (OPL; inner boundary) and at the level of Bruch's membrane (BM; outer boundary). Blood flow between these segmentation lines were projected in the OCT angiogram. An "artifact removal" toggle function within the software was used to subtract the retinal vessel shadowing from the OCT angiogram.

DESCRIPTION OF VASCULAR CHANGES USING OCTA

Interpretation of CSCR features in an OCT angiogram requires careful and comprehensive examination, since displacement of retinal layers from their normal levels are frequently present. Therefore, locating scan depth and determining segmentation thickness are essential parts of the analysis. Although CNV can be observed in OCTA by viewing the entire retina, the outer retina, defined as the composition of scans between the BM and OPL contains the segmentation level at which CNV can be located more accurately (Figs 12.1 and 12.2), since normal retinal vessels are not expected at this depth.

CNV related to CSCR is heterogenous with regards to its shape, location and flow and may be particularly suited to being identified on OCTA, since it is rarely associated with massive subretinal hemorrhage that could limit the penetration of OCT signal. On OCTA, the flows have a clear, evident branching with either well-circumscribed (lacy wheel or sea-fan shaped vessels) or poorly-circumscribed (long filamentous vessels) appearance. Location with respect to the RPE and BM can be done with manual adjustment of the segmentation lines.

Different therapeutic modalities are available to treat CSCR associated or not to CNV and some vascular effects secondary to these treatments can be also observed by using OCTA. In eyes recently treated with anti-vascular endothelial growth factor (VEGF), fragmentation and fading of flow signs occur in the CNV area (Fig. 12.3). Long-term effects of PDT such as choroidal vascular remodeling and recanalization of occluded vessels and choriocapillary occlusion[10-12] may confound the accurate determination of CNV size in CSCR treated eyes (Fig. 12.4).[12]

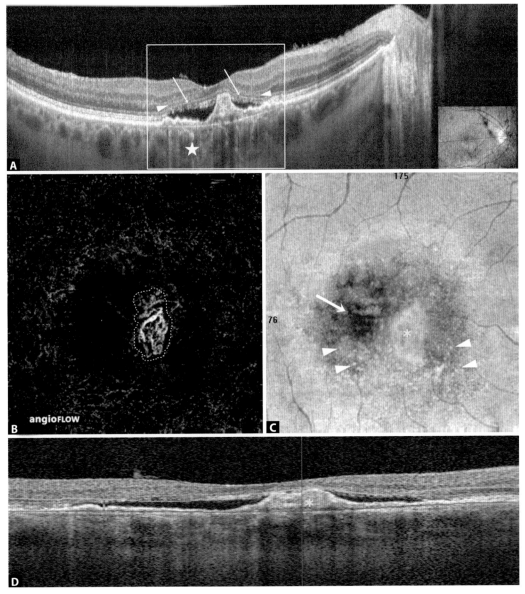

Figs 12.1A to D: Images obtained using the Angiovue optical coherence tomography angiography (OCTA) software of the RTVue XR Avanti (Optovue, Inc., Fremont, CA) of the right eye of a 63-year-old Caucasian woman with chronic central serous chorioretinopathy associated with a type 1 choroidal neovascularization (CNV). (A) A 12 mm high-definition OCT B-scan at the fovea shows a fibrovascular retinal pigment epithelial detachment (RPED) surrounded by subretinal fluid and shallow RPE elevations. Classical features of central serous chorioretinopathy as thickened choroid (yellow star), elongation of outer segments (arrows) and shortening of outer retina layer (arrowheads) are observed. (B) Protocol 3 x 3 mm of an OCT angiogram at the outer retina level shows the CNV (yellow trace), as well as, retinal vessels shadowing from the superficial and deep retinal vasculature. (C) Three-dimensional reference C-scan at the outer retina level shows relative hyporeflectivity due to serous retinal detachment (arrows) associated with highly reflective dots due to elongated photoreceptor outer segment (arrowheads). The type 1 CNV is shown as an irregular hyperreflective area corresponding to the fibrovascular RPED location (yellow star). (D) Coregistered OCT B-scan shows the RPED (yellow star) and the representation of the outer retina segmentation level which is indicated by two horizontal lines with the inner boundary segmentation corresponding to the outer aspect of the outer plexiform layer (green line) and the outer boundary segmentation line to the Bruch's membrane (red line).

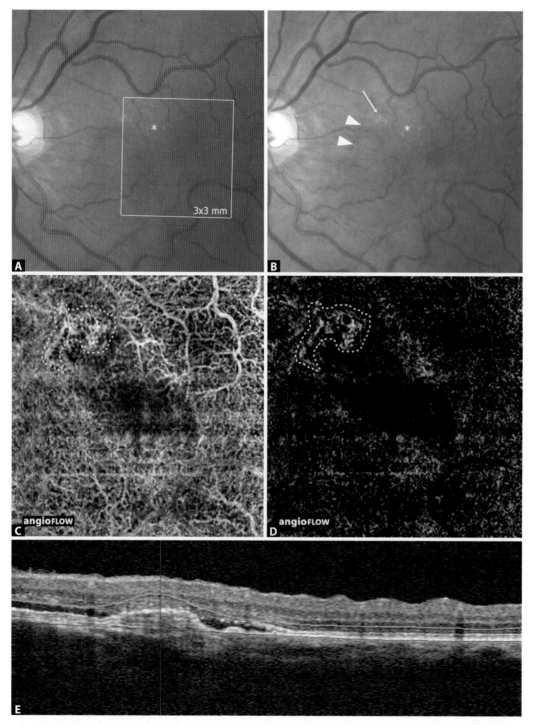

Figs 12.2A to E: Images obtained using the Angiovue optical coherence tomography angiography (OCTA) software of the RTVue XR Avanti (Optovue, Inc., Fremont, CA). Protocol 3 x 3 mm of the left eye of a 70-year-old Caucasian man with chronic central serous chorioretinopathy (CSCR) and choroidal neovascularization (CNV) previously treated with photodynamic therapy (PDT). (A and B) Shallow serous retinal detachment (arrowheads) associated with hard exudates (arrow) surrounding a retinal pigment epithelial detachment (RPED) (*) is observed in color (A) and red free (B) imaging. (C) OCT angiogram depth located at the outer retina level shows the CNV (yellow trace), as well as, positive shadowing from superficial and deep retinal vasculature. (D) Artifact removal toggle function within the software can subtract the retinal vessel shadowing from the *en face* flow image allowing better delineation of the CNV. (E) Coregistered B-scan shows RPED with internal heterogenous hyperreflectivity. Outer retina level is indicated by 2 horizontal lines with the inner boundary segmentation corresponding to the outer aspect of the outer plexiform layer (green line) and the outer boundary segmentation line to the Bruch's membrane (red line)

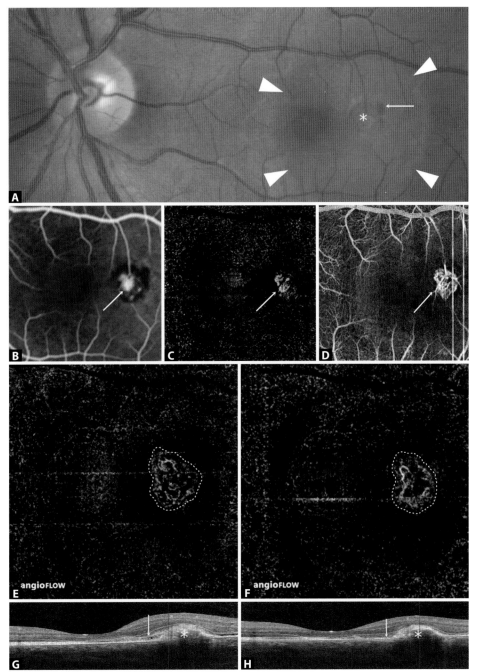

Figs 12.3A to H: Multimodal imaging of the left eye of a 31-year-old Caucasian man with central serous chorioretinopathy complicated with choroidal neovascularization (CNV). (A) Serous retinal detachment (arrowheads) and pigmented retinal pigment epithelial detachment (RPED; *) surrounded by a vestige of subretinal hemorrhage (arrow) were identified at the initial presentation. (B) Fluorescein angiogram showed the CNV as a subretinal area of focal leakage (arrow) surrounded by blockage of the dye secondary to pigment abnormalities and subretinal hemorrhage in this area (*). (C) 3 x 3 mm image obtained using the Angiovue optical coherence tomography angiography (OCTA) software of the RTVue XR Avanti (Optovue, Inc., Fremont, CA). After retinal vessels artifact removal, a CNV presenting well-circumscribed vessels can be identified. (D) 3 x 3 mm image from the same patient acquired in the same date using a prototype swept source OCTA system (Department of Electrical Engineering and Computer Science and Research Laboratory of Electronics, Massachusetts Institute of Technology, Cambridge, MA) showed the CNV slightly different in shape and size. (E) Fifteen days later, the patient received treatment with intravitreal injection of anti-vascular endothelial growth factor in this eye. Pretreatment OCT angiogram from the RTVue XR Avanti OCT angiography showed enlargement of the sizes of the lesion compared to initial presentation. (F) Fifteen days after treatment, vascular flow of the CNV presents a fragmented appearance on the Avanti OCT angiogram, and less anastomoses are visualized in comparison to the pretreatment imaging. (G) Pretreatment coregistered OCT B-scan shows that the delineation of the inner and outer boundaries of outer retina level (green and red lines) included a fibrovascular RPED (*) and subretinal fluid areas (arrow). (H) After treatment, coregistered OCT B-scan shows complete resolution of the subretinal fluid (arrow) and persistence of RPE detachment (*).

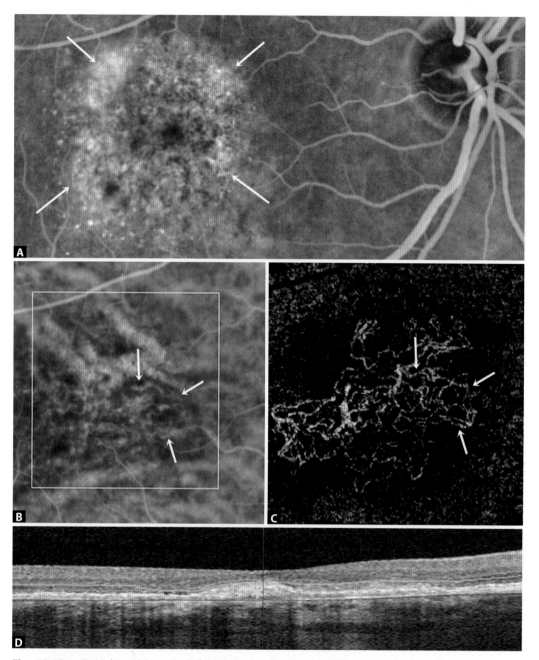

Figs 12.4A to D: Multimodal imaging of the right eye of a 68-year-old Caucasian woman with chronic central serous chorioretinopathy and choroidal neovascularization (CNV) previously treated with photodynamic therapy (PDT). (A) Fluorescein angiography shows stippled hyperfluorescence in the CNV location (arrows). (B) Indocyanine green angiography (ICGA) showed some of the vessels of the CNV associated with multifocal stippled hyperfluorescence. (C) 3 x 3 mm OCT angiogram obtained using the Angiovue optical coherence tomography angiography (OCTA) software of the RTVue XR Avanti (Optovue, Inc., Fremont, CA). After retinal vessels artifact removal, the CNV network can better delineated. Remodeling vessels secondary to PDT treatment may have contributed to CNV appearance on OCTA in this particularly case. Only part of the CNV can be seen with ICGA (yellow and white arrows). (D) Coregistered OCT B-scan shows that delineation of the inner and outer boundaries of the segmentation (green and red lines) included the retinal pigment epithelial detachment (*).

DESCRIPTION OF NONVASCULAR CHANGES USING OCTA

RPEDs related or not to subretinal fluid are frequently found in CSCR eyes. Serous RPED and sub-RPE fibrin do not show any evidence of flow on OCTA (Figs 12.5 to 12.7). However, nonvascular reflecting structures possibly present in the corresponding *en face* structural imaging, such as hard exudates and pigment accumulation, may generate nonvascular "flow" evidence as a result of very small eyes motions or OCT scanning changes (Fig. 12.7).

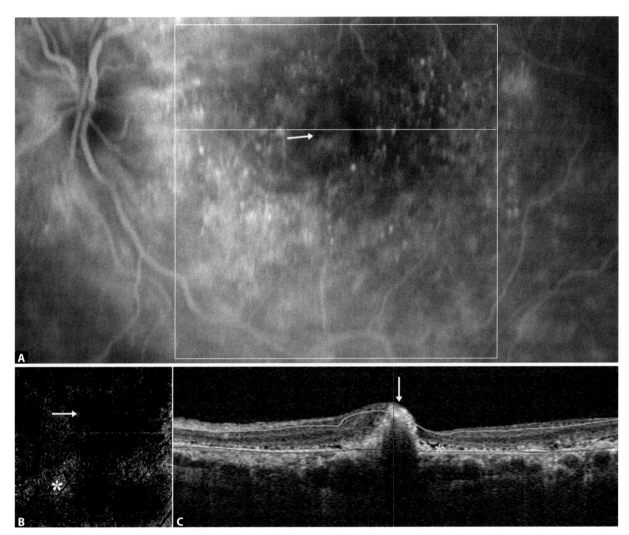

Figs 12.5A to C: Multimodal imaging of the right eye of a 44-year-old Caucasian man with chronic central serous chorioretinopathy with no previous treatment. (A) Fluorescein angiography shows stippled hyperfluorescence in macular area and pooling of dye in the retinal pigment epithelial detachment (RPED) location. (B) 6 x 6 mm image obtained using the Angiovue optical coherence tomography angiography (OCTA) software of the RTVue XR Avanti (Optovue, Inc., Fremont, CA). OCT angiogram after retinal vasculature artifact removal shows absence of abnormal vascular flow and presence of a well-circumscribed area with no vascular flow sign corresponding to shadowing artifact in the topography of the RPED (arrow) in the outer retina. Some areas of choriocapillaris (*) are seen on OCT angiogram secondary to misalignment of outer segmentation line. (C) Coregistered B-scan shows juxtafoveal heterogenous RPED (arrow) surrounded by subretinal fluid (*).

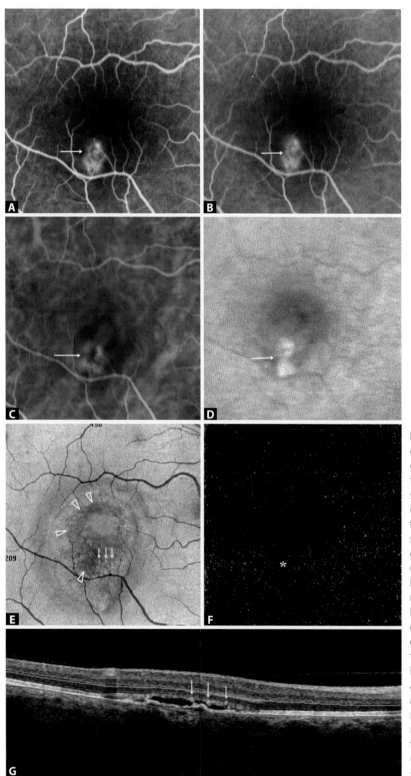

Figs 12.6A to G: Multimodal imaging of the right eye of a 62-year-old Caucasian woman with chronic central serous chorioretinopathy with no previous treatment. (A and B) fluorescein angiography shows subretinal hyperfluorescence in the juxtafoveal area (arrows) with a trace of leakage observed in the late frame (B). (C and D) Indocyanine-green angiography shows focal patchy hyperfluorescence in the inner choroid with leakage observed in the late frame (D). (E) Three-dimensional reference C-scan at outer retina level shows relative hyporeflectivity due to serous retinal detachment (arrowheads) associated with highly reflective dots due to elongated photoreceptor outer segment (yellow arrows). (F) 6 x 6 mm image obtained using the Angiovue optical coherence tomography angiography (OCTA) software of the RTVue XR Avanti (Optovue, Inc., Fremont, CA). OCT angiogram shows absence of abnormal vasculature, and shadowing artifact in the topography of the retinal epithelial detachments (RPED) (*). (G) Co-registered OCT B-scan shows corresponding features of elongated photoreceptor outer segments (yellow arrows) and a shallow heterogeneous RPED surrounded by subretinal fluid.

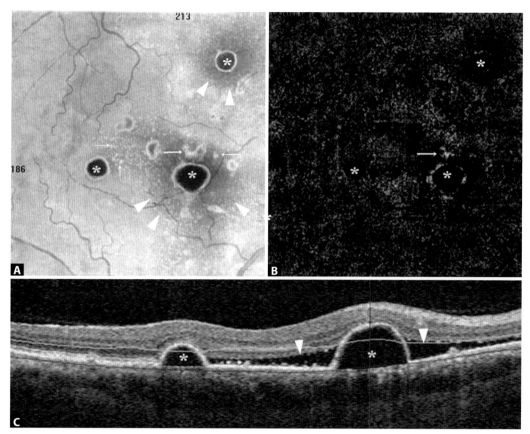

Figs 12.7A to C: Images obtained using the Angiovue optical coherence tomography angiography (OCTA) software of the RTVue XR Avanti (Optovue, Inc., Fremont, CA). 6 x 6 mm of the right eye of a 67-year-old Caucasian man with chronic central serous chorioretinopathy. (A) Three-dimensional reference C-scan at the outer retina level shows relative hyporeflectivity due to serous retinal detachment (arrowheads). Retinal pigment epithelial detachments (RPEDs) are identified as highly reflective rings with low inner reflectivity (*). Highly reflective dots can represent elongated photoreceptor outer segment, RPE villosities abnormalities and/or subretinal fibrinous exudates (arrows). (B) OCT angiogram shows absence of abnormal vascular flow and presence of well-circumscribed areas with no vascular flow sign corresponding to shadowing artifact in the topography of the RPED(*). Nonvascular reflecting structure generating nonvascular "flow" evidence is observed in outer retina segmented C-scan (arrow). (C) Coregistered B-scan shows corresponding RPEDs (*) with low internal reflectivity surrounded by subretinal fluid (arrowheads).

REFERENCES

1. Spaide RF, Campeas L, Haas A, et al. Central serous chorioretinopathy in younger and older adults. Ophthalmology. 1996;103(12):2070-9; discussion 9-80.

2. Guyer DR, Yannuzzi LA, Slakter JS, et al. Digital indocyanine green videoangiography of central serous chorioretinopathy. Arch Ophthalmol. 1994;112(8):1057-62.

3. Liew G, Quin G, Gillies M, Fraser-Bell S. Central serous chorioretinopathy: a review of epidemiology and pathophysiology. Clin Experiment Ophthalmol. 2013;41(2):201-14.

4. De Salvo G, Vaz-Pereira S, Keane PA, et al. Sensitivity and Specificity of Spectral-Domain Optical Coherence Tomography in Detecting Idiopathic Polypoidal Choroidal Vasculopathy. Am J Ophthalmol. 2014.

5. Gilbert CM, Owens SL, Smith PD, Fine SL. Long-term follow-up of central serous chorioretinopathy. Br J Ophthalmol. 1984;68(11):815-20.

6. Gomolin JE. Choroidal neovascularization and central serous chorioretinopathy. Can J Ophthalmol. 1989;24(1):20-3.

7. Ahlers C, Geitzenauer W, Stock G, et al. Alterations of intraretinal layers in acute central serous chorioretinopathy. Acta Ophthalmol. 2009;87(5):511-6.

8. Nicholson B, Noble J, Forooghian F, Meyerle C. Central serous chorioretinopathy: Update on pathophysiology and treatment. Surv Ophthalmol. 2013;58(2):103-26.

9. Ferrara D, Mohler KJ, Waheed N, et al. En face enhanced-depth swept-source optical coherence tomography features of chronic central serous chorioretinopathy. Ophthalmology. 2014;121(3):719-26.

10. Schnurrbusch UE, Welt K, Horn LC, et al. Histological findings of surgically excised choroidal neovascular membranes after photodynamic therapy. Br J Ophthalmol. 2001;85(9):1086-91.

11. Dewi NA, Yuzawa M, Tochigi K, et al. Effects of photodynamic therapy on the choriocapillaris and retinal pigment epithelium in the irradiated area. Jpn J Ophthalmol. 2008;52(4):277-81.

12. Chan WM, Lam DS, Lai TY, et al. Choroidal vascular remodelling in central serous chorioretinopathy after indocyanine green guided photodynamic therapy with verteporfin: A novel treatment at the primary disease level. Br J Ophthalmol. 2003;87(12):1453-8.

OCT Angiography Examination of Type 2 Idiopathic Macular Telangiectasia

Ching J Chen, Matthew Olson, Royce Chen

INTRODUCTION

Macular telangiectasia is a slowly progressive retinal disease with ectasis of the perifoveal vessels and loss of both inner and outer retinal tissue, that can eventually lead to cystic change of the macula, or even macular hole formation. Subretinal neovascular membrane (SRNV) can develop in the late stage of the disease and cause significant vision loss.[1-4] Etiology of the disease is not clear, although a neurodegenerative disease involving Müller cells has been postulated.[5-7] The Mac Tel 2 project reported a higher prevalence of systemic ischemic vascular diseases such as hypertension and diabetes mellitus, but they do not appear to be causative factors.[3]

Clinically, it is characterized by telangiectasis of the perifoveal vessels, intraretinal crystalline deposits, cystic changes, macular hole, pigment clumping, right-angled venules, SRNV, macular edema, subretinal hemorrhage, and macular disciform scar formation.[1,2,7,8]

The disease was originally reported by Donald Gass in 1968.[9] He offered the first classification and staging of the disease in 1982[10] based on the observation of the clinical course of the disease, fundus examination and fluorescein angiography (FA). Subsequently, he revised the classification with Blodi in 1993.[11] In an attempt to simplify the classification system, Yannuzzi recommended dividing the disease to only two types, namely Mac Tel 1 (aneurysmal telangiectasia), and Mac Tel 2 (perifoveal telangiectasia). Mac Tel 1 is the original Gass type 1, which is Coat's disease in reality. Gass type 2a and 2b were renamed to Mac Tel 2, the Gass 2b was dropped due to the rarity of the disease.[12]

Although there is no proven treatment in early stages of Mac Tel 2, there were reports of pharmacological therapy with favorable response in proliferative stage of the disease.[1,3,4] It is important for the clinicians to recognize stage 4 and stage 5 diseases and to offer timely treatment.

Diagnosis of Mac Tel 2 is usually based on FA and spectral-domain optical coherence tomography (SD-OCT). However, there are many other newer imaging techniques such as fundus autofluorescence,[13] *En Face* OCT[14] and adaptive optics scanning laser ophthalmoscopy[15] that may provide additional valuable information.

The recent development of OCT angiography allows the clinicians to move one step forward by providing the opportunity to study blood flow in different layers of the retina and choroid without the need for intravenous contrast media. It has quickly become a powerful technology to detect the vascular pathology associated with Mac Tel 2.[16-18] There are many algorithms that can be applied to the OCT instrument to produce a clinically meaningful OCT angiography. We use Split-Spectrum Amplitude-Decorrelation Angiography (SSADA)[19,20] installed in a commercially available SD-OCT machine running at 70 KHz. This allows a high quality OCT angiographic image to be obtained in both 3 × 3 mm and 6 × 6 mm areas.

Clinical findings and staging of the Mac Tel 2 and representative cases:

Diagnosis of early Mac Tel 2 is somewhat difficult due to the lack of significant subjective symptoms and minimal signs of pathology on fundus examination. It can be divided into 5 stages depending on the clinical findings (Table 13.1)

There are typical signs on FA and SD-OCT in the early stage of Mac Tel 2. However, manifestation of the clinical signs can be varied in different stages of the disease, therefore, making the clear-cut delineation of stages somewhat difficult (Table 13.2).

TABLE 13.1: Clinical findings in Mac Tel 2

Stage	Clinical finding
1	Blunting of foveolar reflex, loss of foveal lutein pigment, loss of transparency in the macula with grayish color change
2	Stage 1 changes plus: Telangiectatic vessels at temporal perifoveal area, and extend to nasal area in some cases Crystalline deposits Early macular cystic change
3	Stage 2 changes plus: Pigment clumping Mild distortion of perifoveal vessels Right-angled venules Lamellar or full thickness macular hole Vascular ingrowth under internal limiting membrane and extending to the foveal avascular zone (FAZ)
4	Stage 3 changes plus: Subretinal neovascular membrane (SRNV) Subretinal or intraretinal hemorrhage Subretinal exudate Retinal edema
5	Stage 4 changes plus: Disciform fibrovascular membrane

TABLE 13.2: Clinical signs of Mac Tel 2 in fluorescein angiography and SD-OCT

Stage/Imaging	Fluorescein angiography	SD-OCT
Stage I	• Hyper-autofluorescent • Low-grade deep fluorescein leakage temporal to the foveola	• Cystic tissue defect with hyporeflective cavities involving the inner retinal layer initially • Disruption of ellipsoid zone
Stage 2	• Fluorescein filling of the temporal perifoveal telangiectatic capillaries • Fluorescein leakage: temporal sector predominantly in early phase, then diffuse hyperfluorescence in late phase	All findings of stage 1 plus: • Hyporeflective cystic cavity may enlarge to involve the inner and outer retina • Crystalline spots with increased reflectivity of the inner retinal layer
Stage 3	All stage 2 findings plus • Capillary ingrowth into FAZ with fluorescein leakage involving the center of fovea in some cases • Dilated right-angled venules • Fluorescein blockage by pigment clumps	All findings of stage 2 plus: • Pigment clumps with increased reflectivity at intra- or subretinal space • Optical shadowing effects by the pigment • Lamellar or full thickness macular hole
Stage 4	All stage 3 findings plus • Fluorescein leakage from SRNV	All findings of stage 3 plus: • Destruction of RPE • Increased reflectivity from SRNV
Stage 5	• Fluorescein leakage from SRNV • Fluorescein staining of the disciform lesion	All findings of stage 3 plus: • Thinning of outer retina • Increased reflectivity from large disciform lesion

OCT angiography with *en face* scanning capability can detect specific vascular changes in the different layers of the retina, and hence is very-well suited for the study of Mac Tel 2. The Angiovue software of the current Optovue SD-OCT produces 4 *en face* OCT angiograms in preselected tissue slabs. Segmentation settings of the tissue slabs in the OCT angiography are shown in Figures 13.1A to D. The boundaries of these pre-defined slabs can be adjusted manually by the user relative to the computer-segmented reference planes. The reference planes can also be manually adjusted to allow for a more precise determination of the location of the pathology. In order to avoid picking up any vascular flow information above the RPE, we routinely perform manual segmentation on Mac Tel 2 patients with stage 3, 4 and 5 diseases. The upper border of the default "outer retina, RPE slab" is moved down to the RPE to obtain more accurate flow information of the "RPE and sub-RPE slab".

The typical clinical findings on OCT angiography in Mac Tel 2 are listed in Table 13.3.

Case illustration and clinical findings of some common ancillary tests and OCT angiography on patients with Mac Tel 2:

Mac Tel 2, Stage 1

Talangiectatic vascular changes involve the deep retinal capillary plexus, predominantly the temporal perifoveal area (Figs 13.2A to H).

Mac Tel 2, Stage 2

The vascular invasion involves both the superficial and deep retinal capillary plexuses. Depending on the size of the telangiectactic vascular complex and the circulation demand, the patient may develop dilated feeder and draining vessels. Crystalline deposits can occur at the superficial retina (Figs 13.3 and 13.4):

TABLE 13.3: OCT angiographic findings in Mac Tel 2

Stage	OCT-angiography findings
1.	• Normal superficial retinal capillary plexus • Telangiectatic change of the deep retinal capillary plexus predominantly temporal to the foveola
2.	• Mild to moderate ectatic capillaries at the superficial retinal capillary plexus • Significant telangiectasia of the deep retinal capillary plexus temporal to the foveola • Loss of vascular density with capillary drop out at both superficial and deep retinal capillary layers • Irregularity of capillary shape and size at the perifoveal area of both superficial and deep retinal capillary plexuses • Dilated feeder and right-angled draining vessels may be seen
3.	• Foveal avascular zone may become irregular • Further capillary drop out with reduced vascular density at both superficial and deep retinal capillary plexuses • Vascular invasion reaching to the retinal pigment epithelium (RPE) • One or more sets of feeder and draining vessels may be present at superficial and deep retinal plexuses • Vascular in growth into the FAZ may be seen • Pigment clumps with optical shadowing effect may be seen
4.	• Distortion and dragging of vessels at the perifoveal area with irregular shape of FAZ • Blood flow can be detected from the SRNV in the outer retina, RPE and choroidal slabs
5.	• Significant thinning and severe loss of vascular density of the outer retina • Vascular size in the SRNV is large, but the vascular density in the SRNV is low • Blood flow to disciform-fibrovascular membrane can be detected and it may reach the deeper choroid

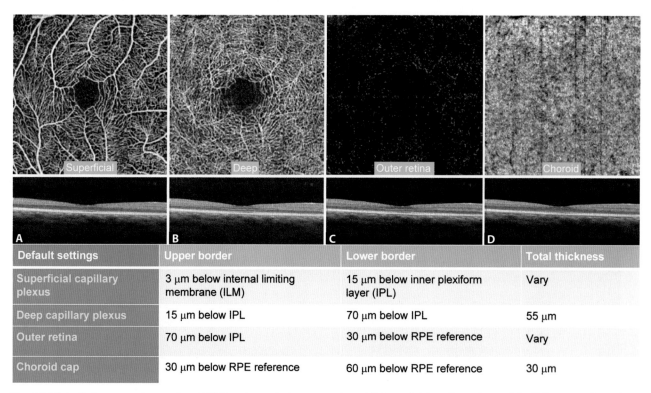

Default settings	Upper border	Lower border	Total thickness
Superficial capillary plexus	3 μm below internal limiting membrane (ILM)	15 μm below inner plexiform layer (IPL)	Vary
Deep capillary plexus	15 μm below IPL	70 μm below IPL	55 μm
Outer retina	70 μm below IPL	30 μm below RPE reference	Vary
Choroid cap	30 μm below RPE reference	60 μm below RPE reference	30 μm

Figs 13.1A to D: Segmentation setting of OCT angiography in a normal eye. (A) Superficial capillary plexus slab. (B) Deep capillary plexus slab. (C) Outer retina slab includes the outer retina and RPE. (D) Choroid cap.

Mac Tel 2, Stage 3

The vasogenic process extends to the internal limiting membrane and the RPE with development of pigment clumping along the dilated vessels. The pigment may migrate to the surface of the retina, or to the subretinal space with distortion of surrounding retinal architecture. More than one set of feeder vessels may be present. Crystalline deposits can occur in the superficial retina (Figs 13.5 to 13.7).

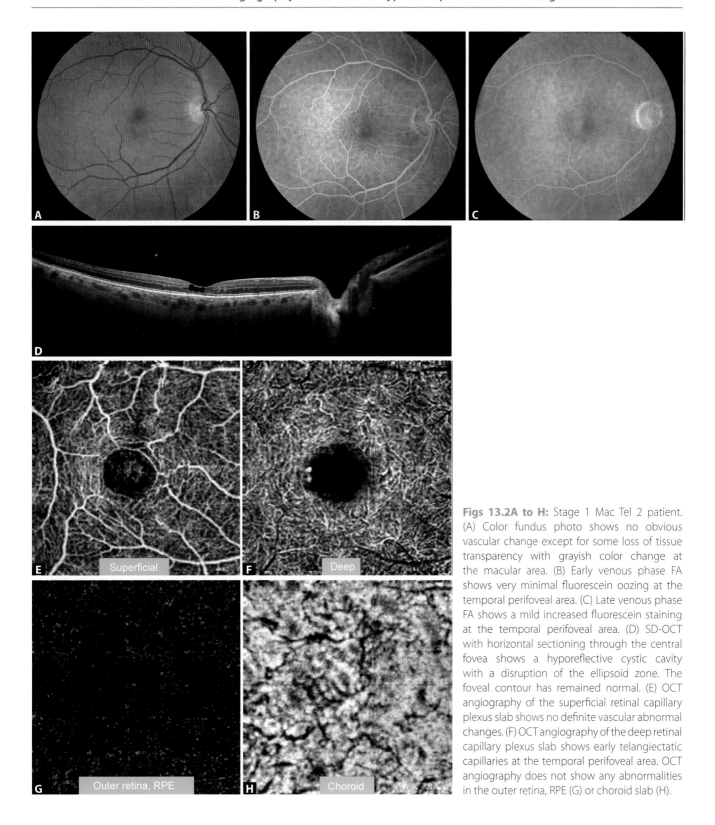

Figs 13.2A to H: Stage 1 Mac Tel 2 patient. (A) Color fundus photo shows no obvious vascular change except for some loss of tissue transparency with grayish color change at the macular area. (B) Early venous phase FA shows very minimal fluorescein oozing at the temporal perifoveal area. (C) Late venous phase FA shows a mild increased fluorescein staining at the temporal perifoveal area. (D) SD-OCT with horizontal sectioning through the central fovea shows a hyporeflective cystic cavity with a disruption of the ellipsoid zone. The foveal contour has remained normal. (E) OCT angiography of the superficial retinal capillary plexus slab shows no definite vascular abnormal changes. (F) OCT angiography of the deep retinal capillary plexus slab shows early telangiectatic capillaries at the temporal perifoveal area. OCT angiography does not show any abnormalities in the outer retina, RPE (G) or choroid slab (H).

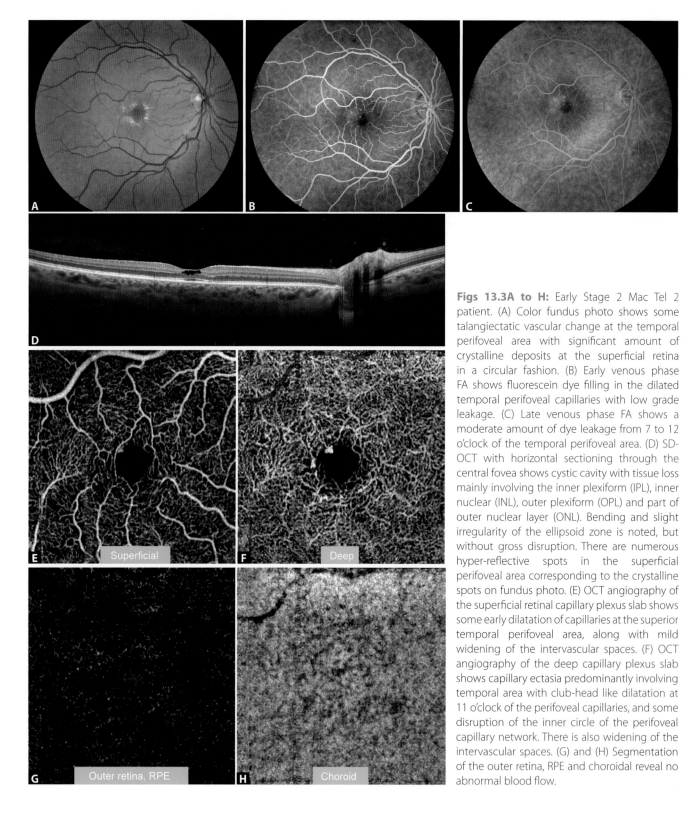

Figs 13.3A to H: Early Stage 2 Mac Tel 2 patient. (A) Color fundus photo shows some talangiectatic vascular change at the temporal perifoveal area with significant amount of crystalline deposits at the superficial retina in a circular fashion. (B) Early venous phase FA shows fluorescein dye filling in the dilated temporal perifoveal capillaries with low grade leakage. (C) Late venous phase FA shows a moderate amount of dye leakage from 7 to 12 o'clock of the temporal perifoveal area. (D) SD-OCT with horizontal sectioning through the central fovea shows cystic cavity with tissue loss mainly involving the inner plexiform (IPL), inner nuclear (INL), outer plexiform (OPL) and part of outer nuclear layer (ONL). Bending and slight irregularity of the ellipsoid zone is noted, but without gross disruption. There are numerous hyper-reflective spots in the superficial perifoveal area corresponding to the crystalline spots on fundus photo. (E) OCT angiography of the superficial retinal capillary plexus slab shows some early dilatation of capillaries at the superior temporal perifoveal area, along with mild widening of the intervascular spaces. (F) OCT angiography of the deep capillary plexus slab shows capillary ectasia predominantly involving temporal area with club-head like dilatation at 11 o'clock of the perifoveal capillaries, and some disruption of the inner circle of the perifoveal capillary network. There is also widening of the intervascular spaces. (G) and (H) Segmentation of the outer retina, RPE and choroidal reveal no abnormal blood flow.

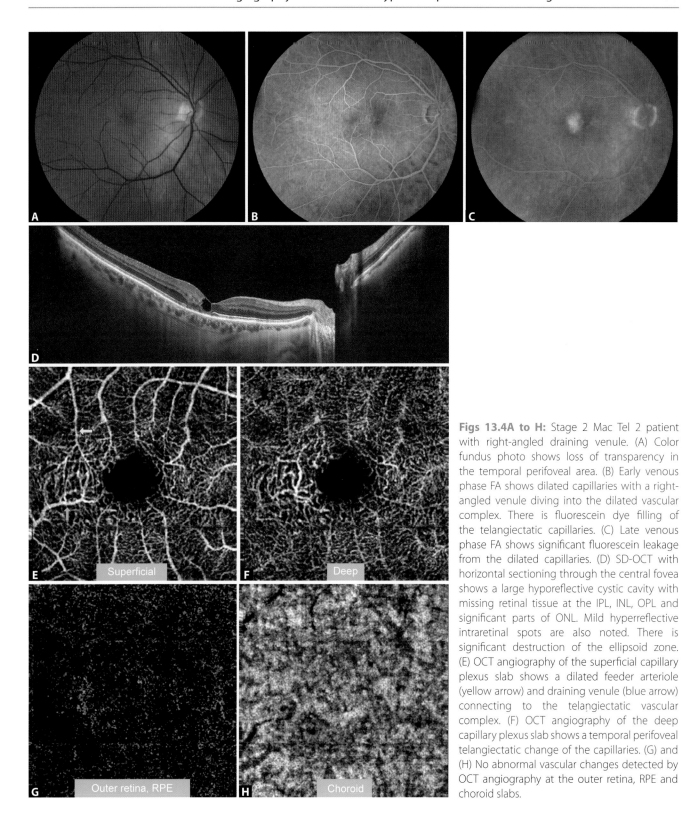

Figs 13.4A to H: Stage 2 Mac Tel 2 patient with right-angled draining venule. (A) Color fundus photo shows loss of transparency in the temporal perifoveal area. (B) Early venous phase FA shows dilated capillaries with a right-angled venule diving into the dilated vascular complex. There is fluorescein dye filling of the telangiectatic capillaries. (C) Late venous phase FA shows significant fluorescein leakage from the dilated capillaries. (D) SD-OCT with horizontal sectioning through the central fovea shows a large hyporeflective cystic cavity with missing retinal tissue at the IPL, INL, OPL and significant parts of ONL. Mild hyperreflective intraretinal spots are also noted. There is significant destruction of the ellipsoid zone. (E) OCT angiography of the superficial capillary plexus slab shows a dilated feeder arteriole (yellow arrow) and draining venule (blue arrow) connecting to the telangiectatic vascular complex. (F) OCT angiography of the deep capillary plexus slab shows a temporal perifoveal telangiectatic change of the capillaries. (G) and (H) No abnormal vascular changes detected by OCT angiography at the outer retina, RPE and choroid slabs.

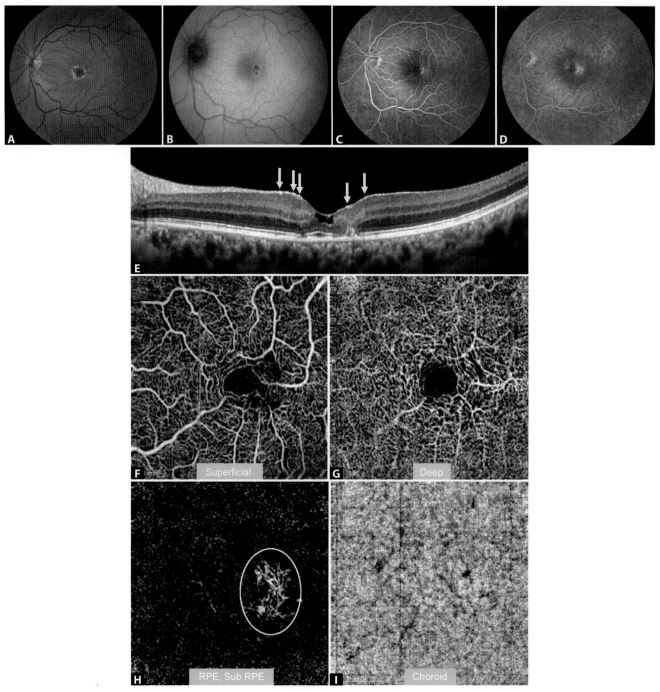

Figs 12.5A to I: Early stage 3 Mac Tel 2 patient with crystalline deposits and mild pigment clumping. The vasogenic process reaches to the RPE. (A) Color fundus photo shows numerous crystalline deposits surrounding the central fovea with mild pigment clumping. (B) Fundus autofluorescence photo highlights two pigment clumps otherwise poorly visualized in the color fundus photo. (C) Early venous phase FA shows a right-angled venule at 3 o'clock in the perifoveal area, and low-grade fluorescein leakage from the temporal telangiectatic capillaries. (D) Late venous phase FA shows moderate fluorescein leakage from the temporal perifoveal dilated vessels, and mild leakage from the nasal perifoveal area. There are also small hypofluorescent spots noted due to fluorescein blockage by the pigment clumps. (E) SD-OCT with horizontal sectioning through the central fovea shows multiple hyperreflective spots on the surface of the retina (yellow arrows) corresponding to the crystalline deposits surrounding the central fovea. A cystic cavity at the fovea involves half the thickness of the central fovea. There is also disruption of the ellipsoid zone. A hyperreflective spot is noted in the outer retina and RPE with mild optical shadowing effect. (F) OCT angiography of the superficial retina slab shows right-angled draining venule at 3 o'clock, and some vascular drop out with disruption of the circular perifoveal capillary net. (G) OCT angiography with deep retina slab shows telangiectatic vascular changes predominantly on the temporal side, but there is also nasal involvement. Significant widening of the intervascular space is noted. (H) Manual segmentation with OCT angiography by moving the upper border of the "default outer retina slab setting" down to the RPE to avoid picking up any flow signal above the RPE, shows the invasion of the telangiectatic vessels reaching to the RPE. (I) There is no choroidal involvement in the choroid slab.

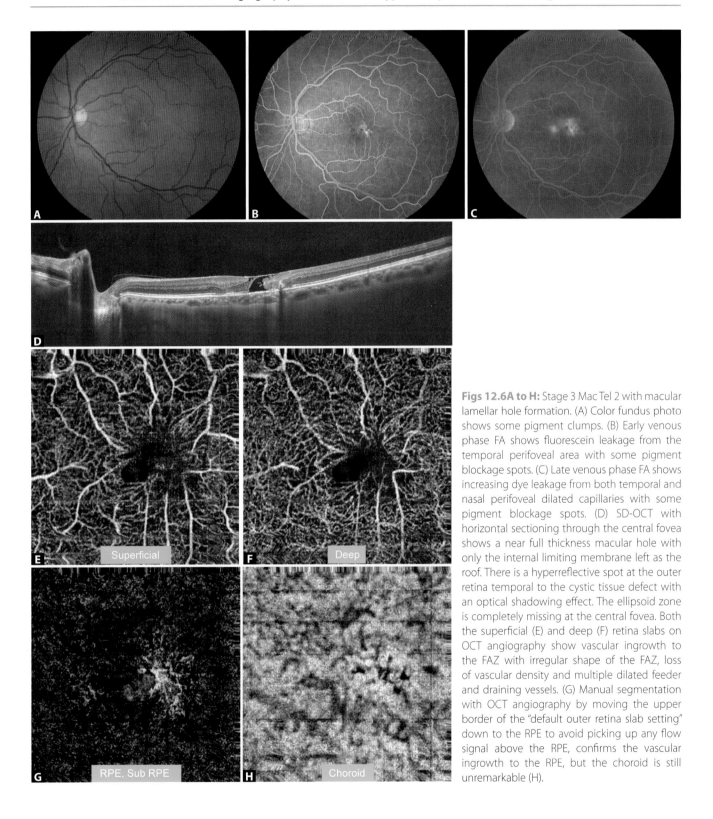

Figs 12.6A to H: Stage 3 Mac Tel 2 with macular lamellar hole formation. (A) Color fundus photo shows some pigment clumps. (B) Early venous phase FA shows fluorescein leakage from the temporal perifoveal area with some pigment blockage spots. (C) Late venous phase FA shows increasing dye leakage from both temporal and nasal perifoveal dilated capillaries with some pigment blockage spots. (D) SD-OCT with horizontal sectioning through the central fovea shows a near full thickness macular hole with only the internal limiting membrane left as the roof. There is a hyperreflective spot at the outer retina temporal to the cystic tissue defect with an optical shadowing effect. The ellipsoid zone is completely missing at the central fovea. Both the superficial (E) and deep (F) retina slabs on OCT angiography show vascular ingrowth to the FAZ with irregular shape of the FAZ, loss of vascular density and multiple dilated feeder and draining vessels. (G) Manual segmentation with OCT angiography by moving the upper border of the "default outer retina slab setting" down to the RPE to avoid picking up any flow signal above the RPE, confirms the vascular ingrowth to the RPE, but the choroid is still unremarkable (H).

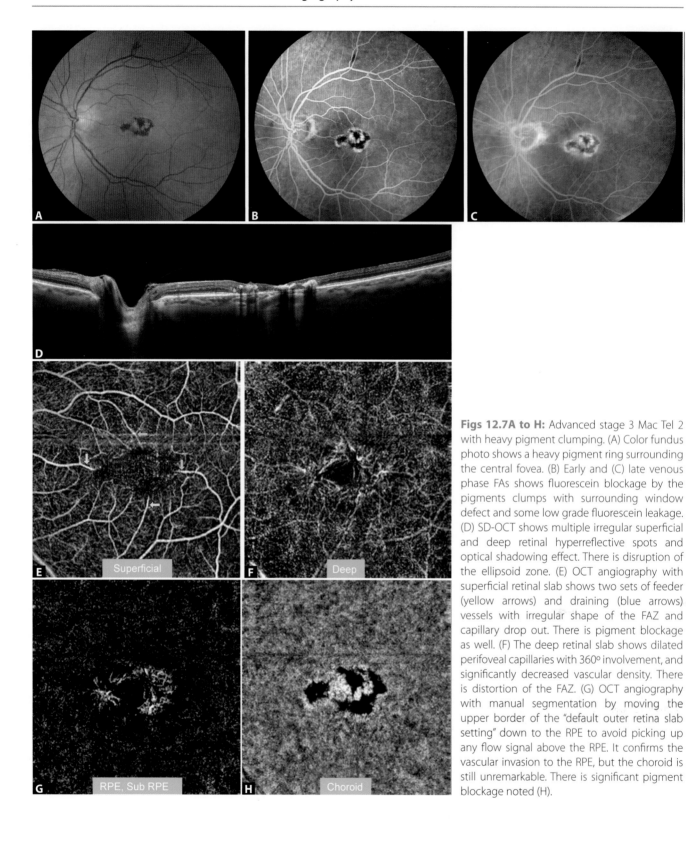

Figs 12.7A to H: Advanced stage 3 Mac Tel 2 with heavy pigment clumping. (A) Color fundus photo shows a heavy pigment ring surrounding the central fovea. (B) Early and (C) late venous phase FAs shows fluorescein blockage by the pigments clumps with surrounding window defect and some low grade fluorescein leakage. (D) SD-OCT shows multiple irregular superficial and deep retinal hyperreflective spots and optical shadowing effect. There is disruption of the ellipsoid zone. (E) OCT angiography with superficial retinal slab shows two sets of feeder (yellow arrows) and draining (blue arrows) vessels with irregular shape of the FAZ and capillary drop out. There is pigment blockage as well. (F) The deep retinal slab shows dilated perifoveal capillaries with 360° involvement, and significantly decreased vascular density. There is distortion of the FAZ. (G) OCT angiography with manual segmentation by moving the upper border of the "default outer retina slab setting" down to the RPE to avoid picking up any flow signal above the RPE. It confirms the vascular invasion to the RPE, but the choroid is still unremarkable. There is significant pigment blockage noted (H).

Mac Tel 2, Stage 4

Stage 4 disease is characterized by vascular proliferation. Subretinal neovascular membrane (SRNV) occurs at this stage. In some cases, the SRNV can penetrate through the RPE to reach the choroid as demonstrated in Figures 13.8 and 13.9.

Mac Tel 2, Stage 5

This is the late proliferative stage of Mac Tel 2 with disciform fibrovascular membrane formation involving the retina, subretina, RPE and choroid as demonstrated in Figure 13.10.

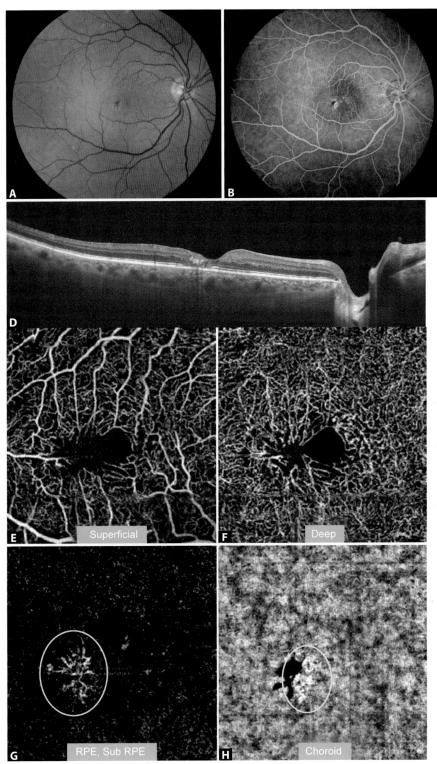

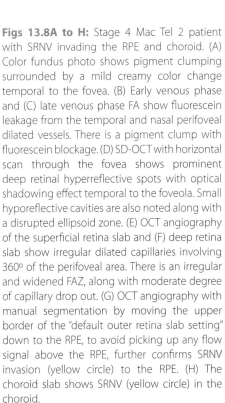

Figs 13.8A to H: Stage 4 Mac Tel 2 patient with SRNV invading the RPE and choroid. (A) Color fundus photo shows pigment clumping surrounded by a mild creamy color change temporal to the fovea. (B) Early venous phase and (C) late venous phase FA show fluorescein leakage from the temporal and nasal perifoveal dilated vessels. There is a pigment clump with fluorescein blockage. (D) SD-OCT with horizontal scan through the fovea shows prominent deep retinal hyperreflective spots with optical shadowing effect temporal to the foveola. Small hyporeflective cavities are also noted along with a disrupted ellipsoid zone. (E) OCT angiography of the superficial retina slab and (F) deep retina slab show irregular dilated capillaries involving 360° of the perifoveal area. There is an irregular and widened FAZ, along with moderate degree of capillary drop out. (G) OCT angiography with manual segmentation by moving the upper border of the "default outer retina slab setting" down to the RPE, to avoid picking up any flow signal above the RPE, further confirms SRNV invasion (yellow circle) to the RPE. (H) The choroid slab shows SRNV (yellow circle) in the choroid.

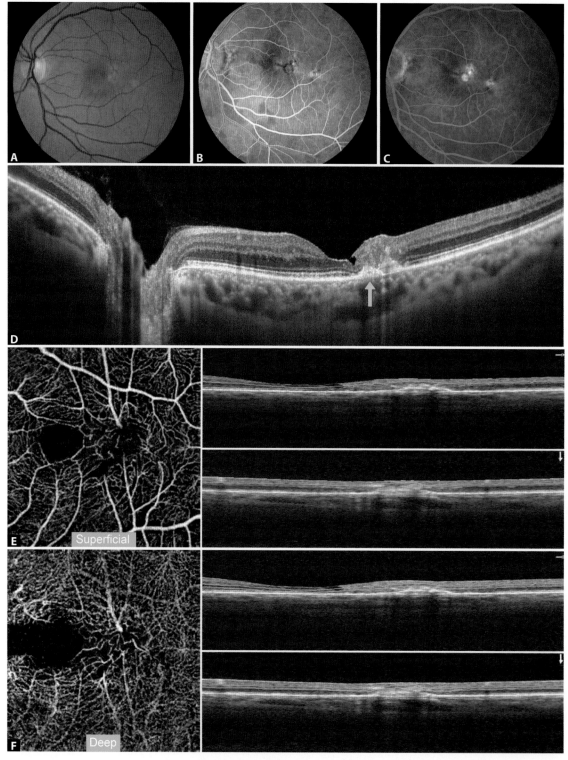

Figs 13.9A to F: Stage 4 Mac Tel 2 patient with SRNV involving the outer retina, RPE and choroid. (A) Color fundus photo shows some pigment clumping next to a SRNV. There is surrounding retinal edema with a slight color change. (B) FA in the early venous phase shows a small bright hyperfluorescent spot superonasal to a slightly larger, moderately hyperfluorescent spot. They are surrounded by a ring of blocked fluorescence. (C) The late venous phase FA shows SRNV with two hyperfluorescent spots and some low-grade fluorescein leakage from the telangiectatic vessels. There is an area with pigment window defect one disc diameter temporal to the macula. (D) SD-OCT shows significantly increased reflectivity from the SRNV (blue arrow) with focal ellipsoid zone and RPE destruction. There is a small hyporeflective cystic cavity at the superficial retina with disrupted ILM. Pigment clumps with increased reflectivity are noted intraretinally temporal to the fovea. (E) OCT angiography with superficial retina slab, and (F) deep retina slab shows significant distortion of the temporal perifoveal vascular pattern, and a significant loss of vascular density. A dilated draining venule is noted. SRNVs (yellow circles) are detected in both the outer retina and RPE.

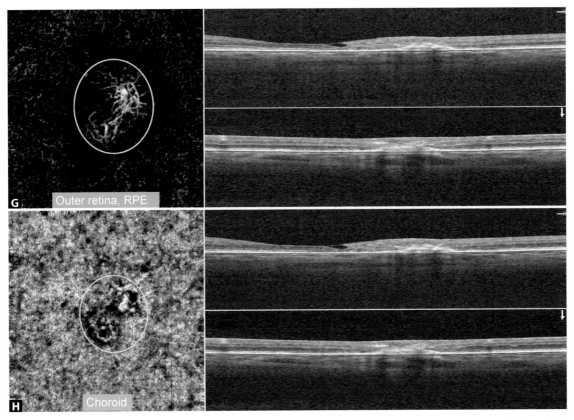

Figs 12.9G and H: Stage 4 Mac Tel 2 patient with SRNV involving the outer retina, RPE and choroid. (G) and choroid (H) slabs. Segmentation line location is shown by horizontal and vertical OCT images (respective arrows) on to the right side of the angioflow images.

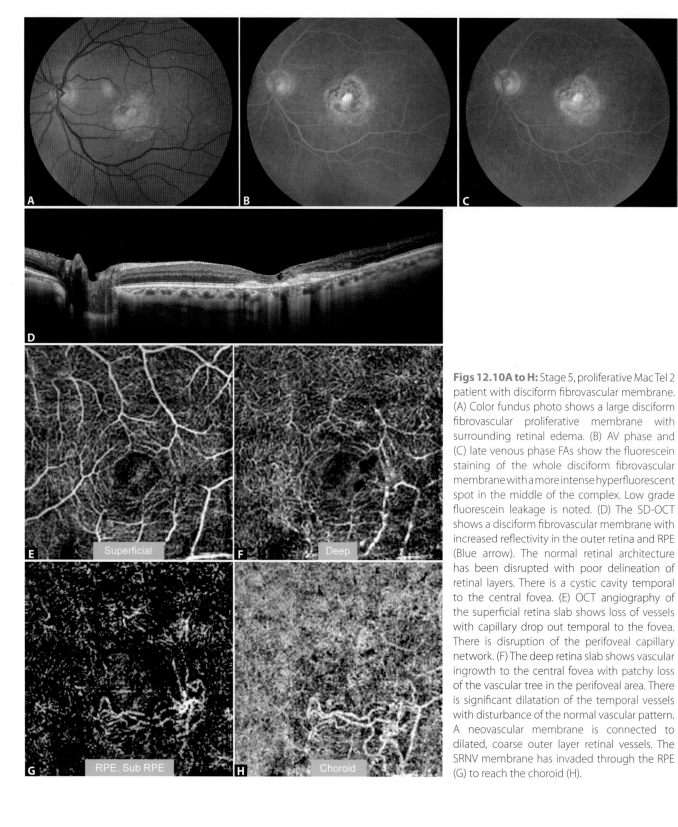

Figs 12.10A to H: Stage 5, proliferative MacTel 2 patient with disciform fibrovascular membrane. (A) Color fundus photo shows a large disciform fibrovascular proliferative membrane with surrounding retinal edema. (B) AV phase and (C) late venous phase FAs show the fluorescein staining of the whole disciform fibrovascular membrane with a more intense hyperfluorescent spot in the middle of the complex. Low grade fluorescein leakage is noted. (D) The SD-OCT shows a disciform fibrovascular membrane with increased reflectivity in the outer retina and RPE (Blue arrow). The normal retinal architecture has been disrupted with poor delineation of retinal layers. There is a cystic cavity temporal to the central fovea. (E) OCT angiography of the superficial retina slab shows loss of vessels with capillary drop out temporal to the fovea. There is disruption of the perifoveal capillary network. (F) The deep retina slab shows vascular ingrowth to the central fovea with patchy loss of the vascular tree in the perifoveal area. There is significant dilatation of the temporal vessels with disturbance of the normal vascular pattern. A neovascular membrane is connected to dilated, coarse outer layer retinal vessels. The SRNV membrane has invaded through the RPE (G) to reach the choroid (H).

CONCLUSION

SSADA based OCT angiography can provide excellent retinal vascular imaging in Mac Tel 2 patients without the need for contrast media. The *en face* scanning capability allows segmentation at the desired level to detect vascular flow information at the specific tissue depth. Because of its unique vascular imaging capabilities, OCT angiography with the SSADA algorithm is a powerful new tool for the clinical study of Mac Tel 2 patients.

REFERENCES

1. Wu L, Evans T, Arevalo JF. Idiopathic macular telangiectasia type 2 (idiopathic juxtafoveolar retinal telangiectasis type 2A, Mac Tel 2). Surv Ophthalmol. 2013 Nov-Dec;58(6):536-59.

2. Nowilaty S, Al-shamsi H, Al-khars W. Idiopathic juxtafoveolar retinal telangiectasis: A current review. Middle East. Afr J Ophthalmol 2010 Jul-Sep;17(3):224-41.

3. Issa PC, Gillis MC, Chew EY, et al. Macular telangiectasia type 2. Progress in Retinal and Eye Research. 2013;34:49-77.

4. Yannuzzi LA. Macular telangiectasia. In: Yannuzzi LA, ed. The Retinal Atlas. Philadelphia, PA, Elsevier Saunders. 2010;422-9.

5. Gass JD. Muller cell cone, an overlooked part of the anatomy of the fovea centralis: hypotheses concerning its role in the pathogenesis of macular hole and foveomacular retinoschisis. Arch Ophthalmol. 1999;117:821-3.

6. Powner MB, Gillies MC, Tretiach M, et al. Perifoveal Muller cell depletion in a case of macular telangiectasia type 2. Ophthalmology. 2010;117:2407-16.

7. Cohen SM, Cohen ML, El-Jabali F, et al. Optical Coherence tomography findings in nonproliferative group 2a idiopathic juxtafoveal retinal telangiectasis. Retina. 2007;27:59-66.

8. Chew E. Perifoveal telangiectasis. In: Ryan SJ, ed. Retina. Philadelphia, PA, Elsevier Mosby. 2006;1409-15.

9. Gass JD. A fluorescein angiographic study of macular dysfunction secondary to retinal vascular disease. V Retinal telangiectasis. Arch Ophthalmol. 1968;80:592-605.

10. Gass JD, Oyakawa RT. Idiopathic juxtafoveal retinal telangiectasis. Arch Ophthalmol. 1982;100:769-80.

11. Gass JD, Blodi BA. Idiopathic juxtafoveal telangiectasis. Update of classification and follow-up study. Ophthalmology. 1993;100:1536-46.

12. Yannuzzi LA, Bardal AM, Freund KB, et al. Idiopathic macular telangiectasia. Arch Ophthalmol. 2006;124:450-60.

13. Wong WT, Forooghian F, Majumdar Z, et al. Fundus autofluorescence in type 2 idiopathic macular telangiectasia: Correlation with optical coherence tomography and microperimetry. Am J Ophthalmol. 2009: 148:573-83.

14. Mauget-Faysse M, Wolff B, Basdekidou, et al. *En Face* optical coherence tomography in idiopathic macular telangiectasia. In: Lumbroso B, Huang D, Romano A, et al. (Eds). Clinical *En Face* OCT atlas. New Delhi, London, Philadelphia, Jaypee Brother Medical Publishers. 2013:235-53.

15. Ooto S, Hangai M, Takayama K, et al. High-resolution photoreceptor imaging in idiopathic macular telangiectasia type 2 using adaptive optics scanning laser ophthalmoscopy. Inves Ophthalmol Vis Sci. 2011; 52(8):5541-50.

16. Lumbroso B, Rispoli M. Savastano, et al. Clinical application: Aspects of OCT SSADA angiography in eye disorders. In: Lumbroso B, Huang D, Jia Y, et al. (Eds). Clinical Guide to Angio-OCT. New Delhi, London, Philadelphia, Jaypee Brother Medical Publisher, 2015:1-4.

17. Spaide RF, Klancnik Jr JM, Cooney M. Retinal vascular layers in macular telangiectasia type 2 imaged by optical coherence tomographic angiography. JAMA Ophthalmology; published online 2014, October 9.

18. Thorell WR, Zhang Q, Huang Y, et al. Swept-Source OCT Angiography of Macular Telangiectasia Type 2, Ophthalmic Surgery, Lasers, and Imaging Retina. 2014;45(5):369-80.

19. Jia Y, Tan O, Tokayer J, Potsaid B, et al. Split-spectrum amplitude-decorrelation angiography with optical coherence tomography. Opt Express. 2012;20(4):4710-25.

20. Tokayer J, Jia Y, Dhalla A, Huang D. Blood flow velocity quantification using split-spectrum amplitude-decorrelation angiography with optic coherence tomography. Biomed Opt Express. 2013;4(10):1909-24.

OCT Angiography of Vascular Occlusions

Marco Rispoli, Bruno Lumbroso, Maria Cristina Savastano

RETINAL VEIN OCCLUSIONS
Fluorescein Angiography

Vein occlusions, as seen with fluorescein angiography, present two basic alterations: Anomalies in vessel permeability and retinal ischemia.[1]

Vein occlusions can, therefore, be subdivided into:

- Edematous occlusions: The abnormal permeability of the vessels causes retinal edema, hemorrhages and exudates with intraretinal fluid leakage (Fig. 14.1)

- Ischemic occlusions: The ischemia leads to the appearance of cotton-wool exudates and highlights hypofluorescent sectors for hypo- or non-perfusion of the capillaries (Fig. 14.2)

- Mixed edematous ischemic occlusions: As a consequence of a vein occlusion, mixed forms may occur with both edematous and ischemic components, with at times one form prevailing over the other (Fig. 14.3)

- Vein occlusions in young patients: They usually regress spontaneously (Fig. 14.4).

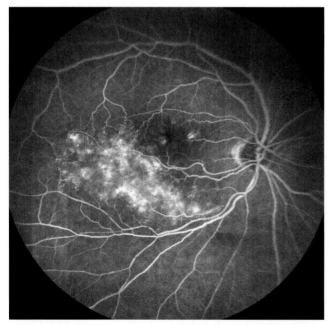

Fig. 14.1: Fluorescein angiography. Edematous type of a branch vein occlusion: this angiographic image shows intense staining of the occluded area that prevents visualization of the underlying vascular network. The fluorescein leaks inside the retina.

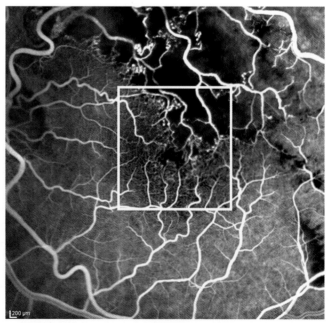

Fig. 14.2: Fluorescein angiography. Ischemic branch vein occlusion. The area of hypofluorescence is evident for lack of perfusion in the occluded area. Truncated vessels and early shunts can be seen. (*Courtesy:* Luca Di Antonio).

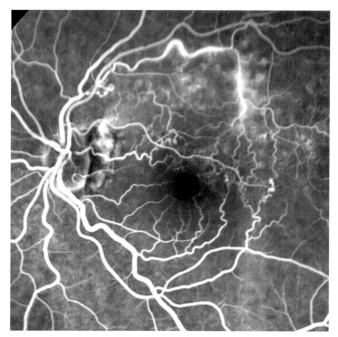

Fig. 14.3: Fluorescein angiography. Branch vein occlusion. Areas with reduced perfusion coexist alongside areas with late fluorescein staining. Notice the alteration of the vascular fluorescein where the staining makes it impossible to assess the size of the vessel.

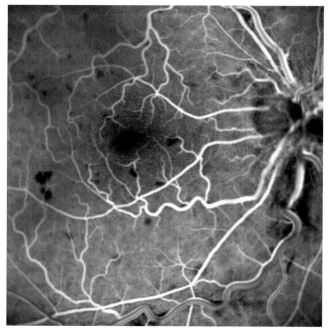

Fig. 14.4: Fluorescein angiography. Vein occlusion in a young patient. Even though the vessel course is altered, there is marked congestion and hemorrhagic masking associated with hyperfluorescence of the optic disc; the prognosis of this syndrome is usually good.

Evolution

Various factors regulate the evolution of vein occlusions.[2]

1. Age-related factors and cause of the obstruction
2. Extent of the obstruction: This depends on the morphology of the lamina cribrosa and on the possibility of anastomoses of the optic-ciliary vessels.

Fluorescein angiography was necessary for the diagnosis and study of the evolution of vein occlusions and for determining the type of treatment. An exploration of all the peripheral quadrants makes it possible to identify all the lesions that may appear during the disease. FA also makes it possible to assess the presence, if any, of retinal and iris neovascularization that precedes neovascular glaucoma.

The prognosis of untreated vein occlusions is always negative except for the juvenile forms that usually regress spontaneously. New treatment has improved recently venous occlusion prognosis. In edematous capillary disorders where blood stasis and vasodilation prevail, there is a quick formation of cystoid macular edema with severe visual impairment.

In the forms with ischemic capillary diseases instead, nonperfusion prevails with involvement of the arterioles. New vessels may appear with dangerous hemorrhages. In some cases, the nonperfusion develops neovascular glaucoma.

OCT Angiography Features in Vein Occlusions

All the OCT angiography figures in this chapter were obtained with a commercial spectral domain OCT device, (SD-OCT, XR Avanti "Angiovue", Optovue, Fremont, CA) imaging at 840 nm wavelength. Two automated segmentation lines were manually

tuned to be located at desired position. Blood flow between these segmentation lines was registered. An artifact removal function was used to eliminate the retinal vessel shadowing.

There is a sharp visual difference between fluorangiography and angio-OCT.

Superficial Vascular Plexus

In vein occlusions, we see changes in the structure of the superficial plexus especially in macular ischemia. The vascular signal (flow) is not linear but has focal deviations, the wall thickness is not regular but shows focal segmentation and lumen narrowing; the vessels course shows abrupt interruptions with some dilation around the avascular foveal area that appears to be widened with respect to healthy individuals. Vessel flow can be segmented.

The vascular network is seen more sharply, and the arteriovenous anastomoses and vascular loops are easier to see. We can observe features which are not possible to observe in fluorangiography because dye leakage hides them in the intermediate and later stages of the examination. Retinal hemorrhages are visible as masked areas but they are much less evident than in fluorangiography.

Retinal edema areas cannot be seen because there is no dye staining or leakage. However, in case of edema we observe a widening and distortion of the capillary network meshes and a decrease in the sharpness of the widened capillaries.

Deep Vascular Plexus

The deep vascular plexus shows more lesions than the superficial plexus. It varies significantly with considerable differences mainly in the ischemic areas. Capillaries distribution is irregular with various changes in vessel course in non-perfused zone. The wall vessels are thicker in the pathologic area; the vessels course shows multiple shunts along various retinal planes.

BRANCH VEIN OCCLUSION
Fluorescein Angiography Aspects

Branch vein occlusions may be ischemic, edematous or mixed and they occur in districts that are more limited compared to the central form.[3]

It is important to locate the site of the occlusion by means of fluorescein angiography.

The occlusion usually occurs at an arterovenous crossing and the venous wall is intensely stained by the fluorescein. There may also be fluorescein leakage. In the occluded area, the capillaries are visibly dilated and tortuous with fluorescein leakage. Often, the occluded area is covered with exudates and hemorrhages. If the macular and perimacular circulation is involved, visual loss occurs right from the earlier stages of the disorder.

In the edematous form, at the periphery of the affected area, collateral vessels may be observed with arterovenous anastomoses and capillary dilatation. Any interruption of the perifoveal arch will have a negative prognosis. At some anastomoses, an inversion of the venular circulation may be observed.

In the ischemic or mixed forms of branch vein occlusion, new vessels may appear at the edges of the occluded area. In these cases, laser treatment of the nonperfused areas may prevent hemorrhaging and in some cases also neovascular glaucoma.

OCT-Angiography Aspects

In eyes affected by vein occlusion, OCT-angiography shows the vascular network with evident areas of non-perfusion that correspond to the areas of non-perfusion visible on the fluorescein angiography. These areas can be easily seen because there is no "masking" caused by fluorescein leakage in the intermediate and late stages.

Superficial Plexus

An increase in the size of some capillaries may be observed while others have a narrower lumen. The ensuing configuration is a coarse network of vessels with meshes of irregular shapes and a grayish background (Fig. 14.5).

Vascular details are sharper than can be seen with fluorescein angiography as, for instance, the arteriovenous anastomoses and the vascular loops.

The vascular texture varies in aspect from fine to coarse. Often the capillaries within the non-perfused areas are truncated, with abrupt interruptions, or there are arteriovenous anastomoses, and connections to the capillary layers of the deep vascular network at the level of the inner nuclear layer (Fig. 14.6).

The areas of retinal edema can be easily identified because there is no staining, but a widening and distortion of the meshes of the capillary network can be noticed as well as a decrease in the sharpness of the dilated capillaries.

When the fluorescein angiography shows vessel walls stained with fluorescein, OCT-angiography instead shows a very weak flow (corresponding to the lumen itself) surrounded by a

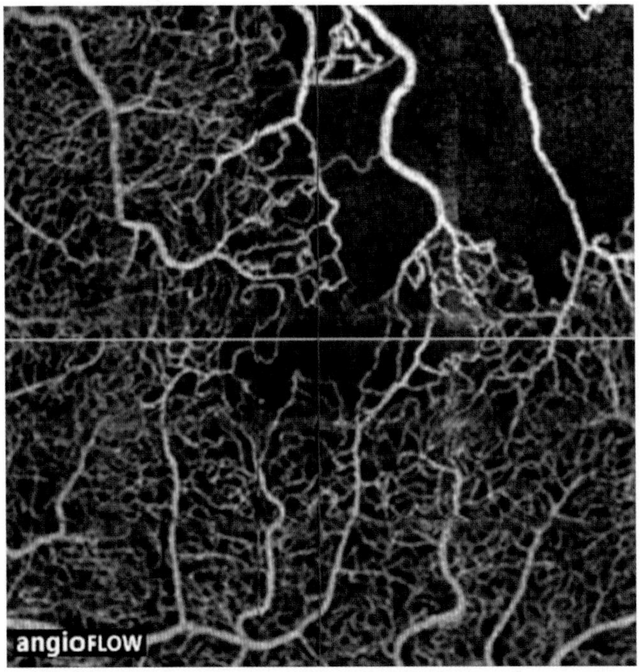

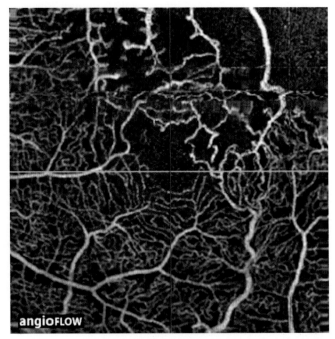

Fig. 14.5: OCT-angiography of ischemic area in a vein occlusion. The ischemic area is clearly perceived as absence of flows in the occluded area. Note the initial formation of anastomoses and collateral circulation at the edges of the ischemic area. (*Courtesy:* Luca Di Antonio).

Fig. 14.6: Truncated vessels, with abrupt interruptions in the areas of non-perfusion in a vein occlusion seen with OCT-angiography. Note the absence of collateral branches in the occluded area. (*Courtesy:* Luca Di Antonio).

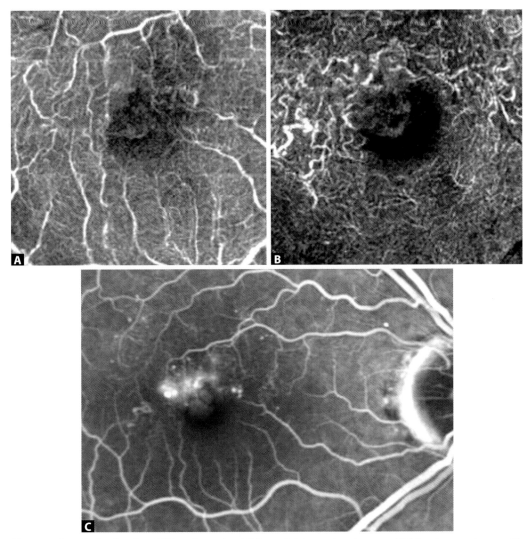

Figs 14.7A to C: Confronting OCT angiography: (A) Superficial vascular plexus and (B) the deeper plexus, with (C) traditional fluorescein angiography. Staining and leakage prevent the observer from seeing a vertical shunt in the temporal macular area, that is associated with marked congestion of the deep vascular plexus.

dark shadow that corresponds to the thickened vessel wall. In this case, therefore, there is a clear cut visual difference between fluorescein angiography and OCT-angiography (Fig. 14.7).

Retinal hemorrhages are visible as masking areas but they are much less evident than can be seen with fluorescein angiography.

In the ischemic areas, the texture of the background may vary from light grey to a greyish granulation.

In the presence of occlusions, changes are observed in the structure of the superficial plexus, especially when there is macular ischemia (Fig. 14.8). In these cases, the outline is not linear but there are focal deviations, and wall thickness is discontinuous with focal segmentation and lumen narrowing; the course of the vessels is abruptly interrupted with terminal

dilatations around the avascular foveal area that appears to be larger than in healthy eyes. The blood flow is segmented along the area affected by the occlusion.

Deep Plexus

The deep plexus is shows variation, mainly in the ischemic areas (Fig. 14.9). Distribution is irregular, with the vessels frequently changing direction in the pathologic area. Vessel walls are thicker in the affected area and the vessels show many shunts between retinal layers. The texture is different in the area where the vascularization is impaired and there is often an increase in pathologic connections between the superficial and deep plexus with marked impairment of vessel size and course (Fig. 14.10).

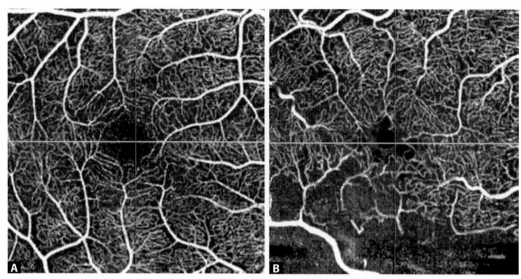

Figs 14.8A and B: (A) Morphological differences of the superficial plexus between a normal eye and (B) in the case of a retinal vein occlusion

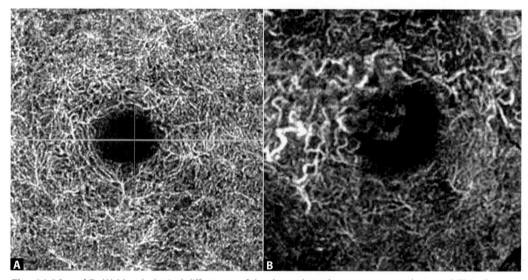

Figs 14.9A and B: (A) Morphological differences of the deep plexus between a normal eye and (B) in the case of a retinal vein occlusion

The affected capillaries shows a slower flow. Vessels appear thin and often with truncated endings at the ischemic areas limits.

BRANCH ARTERY OCCLUSION

In a branch artery occlusion, the superficial network loses some, but not all the collateral branches after the ischemic event. This aspect concerns almost exclusively the superficial vascular plexus. En face imaging features show it better than OCT angiography. At deep network level, capillaries of the deep plexus are intensely upset by arterial occlusion. Important capillary drop out is evident. Some capillaries increase in size while many more are closed. Deep network shows larger and more sparse meshes (Fig. 14.11).

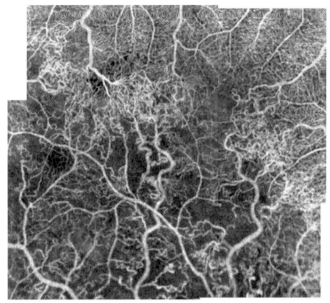

Fig. 14.10A: SLO functional composite of a BRVO case. In this visualization, we can appreciate all overlapping networks. Ischemic areas are clearly seen.

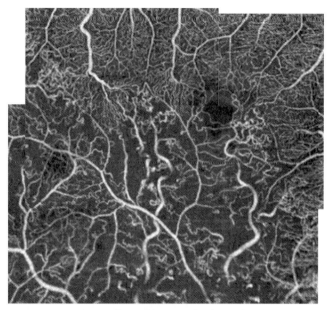

Fig. 14.10B: Angioflow of the superficial vascular plexus. The ischemic tissue shows in some areas a complete flow loss.

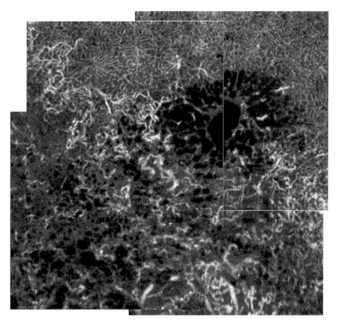

Fig. 14.10C: Angioflow of the deep vascular plexus. Dark areas combine no flow zones and cystic cavities. The superior part of the figure shows normal deep vascular plexus capillaries. The inferior part shows dilated and segmented deep capillaries.

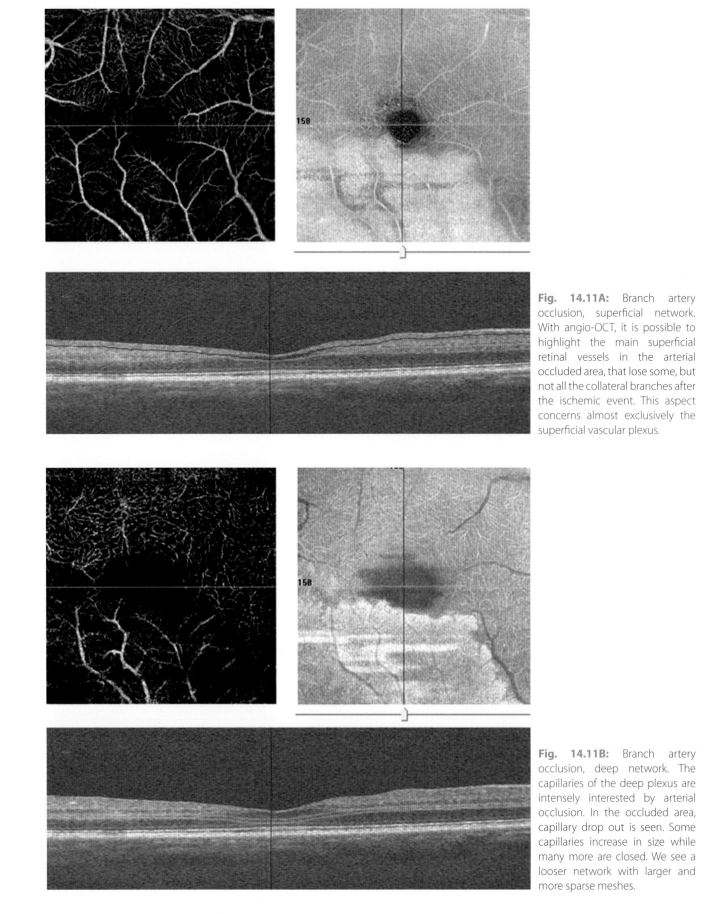

Fig. 14.11A: Branch artery occlusion, superficial network. With angio-OCT, it is possible to highlight the main superficial retinal vessels in the arterial occluded area, that lose some, but not all the collateral branches after the ischemic event. This aspect concerns almost exclusively the superficial vascular plexus.

Fig. 14.11B: Branch artery occlusion, deep network. The capillaries of the deep plexus are intensely interested by arterial occlusion. In the occluded area, capillary drop out is seen. Some capillaries increase in size while many more are closed. We see a looser network with larger and more sparse meshes.

REFERENCES

1. Hayreh SS. Ocular vascular occlusive disorders: natural history of visual outcome. Prog Retin Eye Res. 2014;41:1-25.

2. London NJ, Brown G. Update and review of central retinal vein occlusion. Curr Opin Ophthalmol. 2011;22:159-65.

3. Jaulim A, Ahmed B, Khanam T, Chatziralli IP. Branch retinal vein occlusion: epidemiology, pathogenesis, risk factors, clinical features, diagnosis, and complications. An update of the literature. Retina. 2013;33:901-10.

Diabetic Retinopathy

*Talisa de Carlo, Eric M Moult, WooJhon Choi, Marco Bonini Filho,
James G Fujimoto, Jay S Duker, Nadia K Waheed*

Optical coherence tomography angiography (OCTA) enables highly detailed visualization of microvascular changes associated with diabetes. OCTA of diabetic retinopathy delineates microaneurysms, areas of capillary nonperfusion, retinal capillary tortuosity and dilation, enlargement of the foveal avascular zone (FAZ) and increased perifoveal intercapillary areas, neovascularization of the disc (NVD) and neovascularization of the retina (NVE), as well as choriocapillaris abnormalities.

NONPROLIFERATIVE DIABETIC RETINOPATHY

One of the benefits of OCTA is that it provides three dimensional volumetric data and can therefore be scrolled through or segmented into *en face* slabs, giving a depth resolved image of the retinal and superficial choroidal vasculature that is not possible with standard fluorescein angiography (FA). The Angiovue OCTA software of the commercially available RTVue XR Avanti (Optovue, Inc., Fremont, CA) automatically segments the inner retina into the "superficial" and "deep" vascular plexuses. The superficial inner retina contains the vessels from the retinal nerve fiber layer (RNFL) and the ganglion cell layer (GCL). The deep vascular plexus is a composite of the plexuses at the border of the inner plexiform layer (IPL) and inner nuclear layer (INL) and the border of the INL and outer plexiform layer (OPL). This segmentation provides clinicians with more exact information on which microvascular plexuses are affected in disease. It is also much easier to detect subtle microvascular changes when there are fewer surrounding capillaries to hide the abnormalities. At the same time, it is important to confirm that the automatic segmentation is correct in order to avoid possible artifacts. If the segmentation identifies incorrect layers, vessels may not appear in the *en face* OCTA images, even though they are present. Segmentation is especially challenging in cases with more advanced pathology where the retinal architecture differs significantly from the normal retina. Figure 15.1 shows an example of diabetic macular edema (DME) where *en face* OCTA can be used to visualize vasculature in the presence of edema and cystic changes.

In DME cases, the fluid can be monitored over time in the same fashion as structural *en face* OCT by looking at the deep inner retinal plexus where the majority of the fluid collects (Fig. 15.1).

OCTA shows the retinal vasculature in much higher detail than FA. As seen in Figures 15.2 to 15.4, the microaneurysms appear as focal dilations (yellow circles) or areas of capillary nonperfusion (blue circles). When compared to FA, OCTA can detect most, but not all microaneurysms. However, OCTA also detects microaneurysms not seen using FA. OCTA has a sensitivity threshold and therefore has a slowest detectable flow, which is determined by time between repeated OCT B-scans (the interscan time). Since some microaneurysms may have slower flow than the sensitivity threshold, these microaneurysms are not detected by the OCTA. If the interscan time is increased, sensitivity to visualizing microaneurysms (slow flow lesions) will increase, but there is a tradeoff of increased noise from eye motion.

Detection of microaneurysms is improved with smaller fields of view. Because the same number of A-scans is used to generate both the 3 mm × 3 mm and 6 mm × 6 mm *en face* OCTA images, the 3 mm × 3 mm image will have greater sampling density (A-scans per unit area). Therefore, it is much easier to identify microaneurysms in Figures 15.2 and 15.3, which are 3 mm × 3 mm, than in Figure 15.4, which is 6 mm × 6 mm. Clinically, larger *en face* fields of view would be more useful, but the limited A-scan acquisition speed of the OCT instrument means that there will be a trade off in image quality as the field of view is increased.

Since OCTA visualizes motion contrast from blood flow, it is unable to show leakage, and therefore cannot distinguish

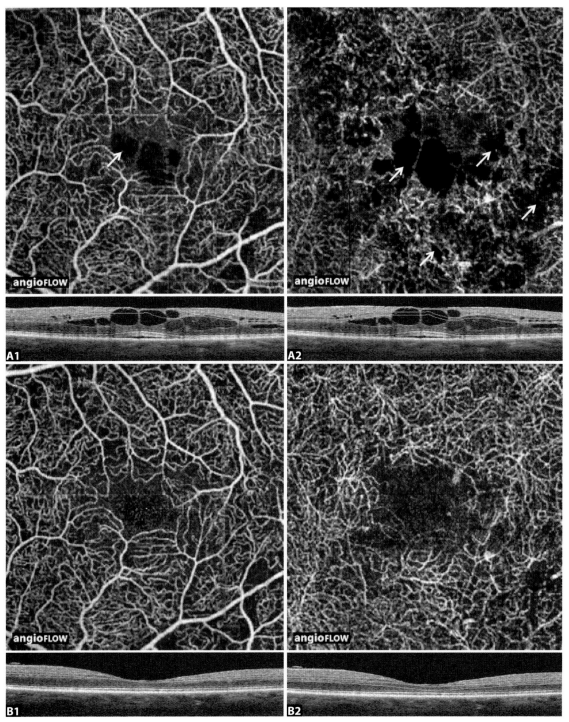

Figs 15.1A and B: Images obtained using the Angiovue optical coherence tomography angiography (OCTA) software of the RTVue XR Avanti (Optovue, Inc., Fremont, CA). (A) 3 mm x 3 mm OCT angiograms and corresponding OCT B-scans of an eye with diabetic macular edema (DME) prior to treatment with intravitreal Aflibercept. (A1) Superficial inner retina showing a few pockets of edema as dark spaces between vessels (example marked by white arrow). The corresponding OCT B-scan demonstrates DME and shows the segmentation between the red and green lines, which is the depth range projected to obtain the *en face* OCTA. (A2) Deep inner retina showing multiple cysts (examples marked by white arrows). The corresponding OCT B-scan demonstrates DME and shows the segmentation of the OCT angiogram as the slab between the two green lines. (B) 3 mm x 3 mm OCT angiograms and corresponding OCT B-scans of the same eye after treatment with intravitreal Aflibercept. (B1) Superficial inner retina shows decreased cystic changes. Corresponding OCT B-scan does not show evidence of DME through that cross-section and shows the segmentation between the red and green lines, which is projected to obtain the *en face* image. (B2) Deep inner retina demonstrates that the edema is mostly improved. The corresponding OCT B-scan does not show evidence of DME through that cross-section and shows the segmentation of the OCT angiogram as the slab between the two green lines.

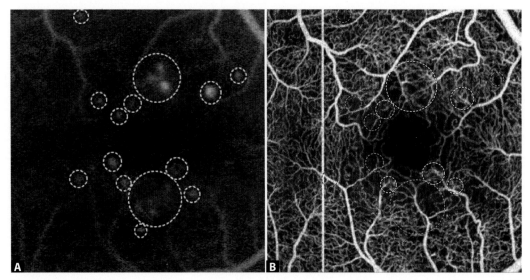

Figs 15.2A and B: Images obtained using a prototype swept source optical coherence tomography (OCT) system at 1,050 nm wavelength (Department of Electrical Engineering and Computer Science, Massachusetts Institute of Technology, Cambridge, MA). (A) Fluorescein angiography (FA) of a diabetic eye cropped to approximately 3 mm x 3 mm. Aneurysms are circled in yellow. (B) 3 mm x 3 mm OCT angiogram of the same eye. Aneurysms that are seen on FA in (A) that are also seen on OCT angiography (OCTA) are circled in yellow. Aneurysms on FA that are seen as areas of capillary nonperfusion on OCTA are circled in blue. Areas where aneurysms are seen on FA, but do not show signs of microaneurysms on OCTA are circled in red.

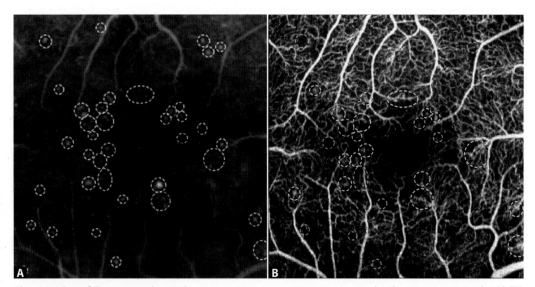

Figs 15.3A and B: Images obtained using a prototype swept source optical coherence tomography (OCT) system at 1,050 nm wavelength (Department of Electrical Engineering and Computer Science, Massachusetts Institute of Technology, Cambridge, MA). (A) Fluorescein angiography (FA) of a diabetic eye cropped to approximately 3 mm x 3 mm. Aneurysms are circled in yellow. (B) 3 mm x 3 mm OCT angiogram of the same eye. Aneurysms that are seen on FA in (A) that are also seen on OCT angiography (OCTA) are circled in yellow. Aneurysms on FA that are seen as areas of capillary nonperfusion on OCTA are circled in blue. Areas where microaneurysms are seen on FA, but not on OCTA are circled in red.

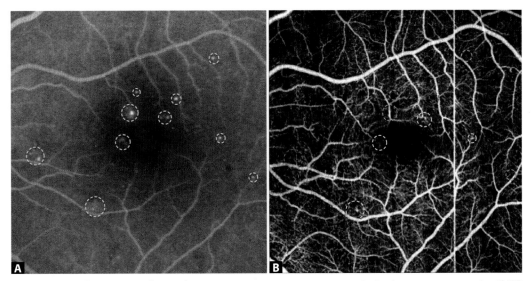

Figs 15.4A and B: Images obtained using a prototype swept source optical coherence tomography (OCT) system at 1,050 nm wavelength (Department of Electrical Engineering and Computer Science, Massachusetts Institute of Technology, Cambridge, MA). (A) Fluorescein angiography (FA) of a diabetic eye cropped to approximately 6 mm x 6 mm. Microaneurysms are circled in yellow. (B) 6 mm x 6 mm OCT angiogram of the same eye. Microaneurysms that are seen on FA in (A) that are also seen on OCT angiography (OCTA) are circled in yellow. Microaneurysms on FA that are seen as areas of capillary nonperfusion on OCTA are circled in blue. Areas where microaneurysms are seen on FA, but not on OCTA are circled in red.

between leaking and nonleaking microaneurysms. However, since OCTA data is generated by repeated OCT B-scans, it also contains intrinsically coregistered volumetric structural data. It is therefore possible to superimpose microvascular images with retinal thickness maps and therefore obtain some indirect information on leakage, Figure 15.5 is an FA in the eye of a patient with diabetic macular edema, showing one leaking microaneurysms and some nonleaking microaneurysms. The OCT angiogram demonstrates these microaneurysms. When the OCT thickness map is superimposed over the OCTA, the pattern of edema is consistent with leakage from one, but not from the other microaneurysms.

An advantage of using OCTA is its highly detailed visualization of retinal capillaries. This makes it much easier to detect microvascular changes, such as telangiectatic vessels and capillary loops, which are difficult to appreciate using other imaging modalities. Most notably, areas of capillary non-perfusion can be readily identified within a dense capillary network. Some of these changes are even present in diabetic eyes considered to have no clinical retinopathy (Fig. 15.6). OCT angiograms of eyes with NPDR demonstrate microvascular changes ranging from mild to severe (Figs 15.7 to 15.13). Some of the changes in eye with mild NPDR closely resemble changes observed in diabetics without clinical retinopathy.

ISCHEMIC DIABETIC MACULOPATHY

The FAZ and perifoveal intercapillary area are progressively enlarged in each stage of diabetic retinopathy (normal eyes to PDR). The ability to accurately delineate these areas is greatly enhanced with the use of OCTA. In Figure 15.14, the FAZ of a normal nondiabetic eye is demarcated in yellow on an OCTA *en face* image (angiogram) and measures 0.16 mm² while the

perifoveal intercapillary area, defined here as areas of non-perfusion at least 0.15 mm² that are continuous with the FAZ, is delineated in white and measures 0.35 mm². Figure 15.15 shows the OCT angiogram of a diabetic eye without retinopathy where the FAZ (yellow) is 0.394 mm² and the perifoveal intercapillary area (white) is 0.881 mm². An OCT angiogram of an eye with non-proliferative diabetic retinopathy (NPDR) is shown in Figure 15.16 alongside an FA. It is not possible to accurately determine the boundaries of the FAZ or perifoveal intercapillary area on the FA. However, on the OCT angiogram, the FAZ (yellow) and perifoveal intercapillary area (white) are clear, measuring at 0.314 mm² and 1.125 mm² respectively. Figure 15.17 shows an OCT angiogram of proliferative diabetic retinopathy (PDR), where the FAZ (yellow) is 0.548 mm² and the perifoveal intercapillary area (white) is 1.899 mm².

PROLIFERATIVE DIABETIC RETINOPATHY

Eyes with PDR show many of the same microvascular changes that are seen in the earlier stages of the disease, but with greater severity. Eyes with PDR may demonstrate large areas of capillary nonperfusion or intraretinal microvascular abnormalities (IRMA) (Figs 15.18 and 15.19).

OCTA can also identify areas of NVE and NVD. The neovascularization is seen as abnormal vessels growing into the vitreous or in the preretinal space. However, it is sometimes difficult to differentiate neovascularization from the inner retinal vasculature using an *en face* OCTA view (Fig. 15.20). In these instances, the coregistered corresponding OCT B-scans can be scrolled through, similar to a macular cube scan, in order to find areas suspicious for neovascularization. These areas

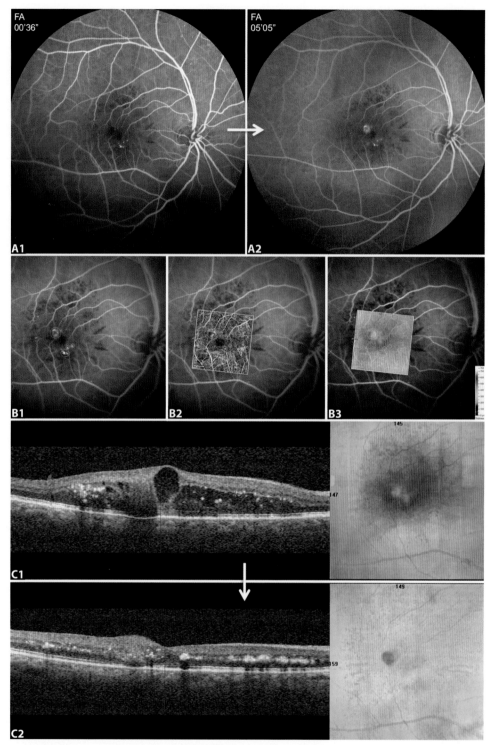

Figs 15.5A to C: Images obtained using the Angiovue optical coherence tomography angiography (OCTA) software of the RTVue XR Avanti (Optovue, Inc., Fremont, CA) of a patient with diabetic retinopathy. (A) Fluorescein angiography (FA) early frame (A1) and late frame (A2) showing that a microaneurysm superotemporal to the fovea is leaking while the microaneurysm inferonasal to the fovea are not leaking. (B1) The microaneurysm are circled in yellow on the zoomed-in late frame of the FA in A. (B2) The 3 mm x 3 mm OCT angiogram is overlain on B1 to show which microaneurysms on the OCT angiogram correspond to those on the FA. (B3) The OCT thickness map from the RTVue XR Avanti is superimposed over (B2) to show that there is thickening due to edema at and around the leaking microaneurysm, while the nonleaking microaneurysms do not show any fluid accumulation. (C1) OCT B-scan and OCT thickness map from the same patient visit in A-B both showing edema. (C2) OCT B-scan and OCT thickness map from the same patient in A-B after approximately three months after two intravitreal injections of Aflibercept. The edema has improved.

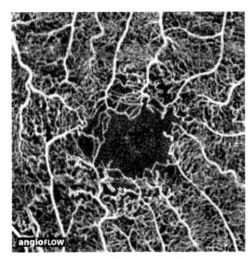

Fig. 15.6: Images obtained using the Angiovue optical coherence tomography angiography (OCTA) software of the RTVue XR Avanti (Optovue, Inc., Fremont, CA). 3 mm x 3 mm OCT angiogram of a diabetic eye without clinical retinopathy showing an enlarged foveal avascular zone (FAZ) and telangiectatic vessels (examples marked by yellow *).

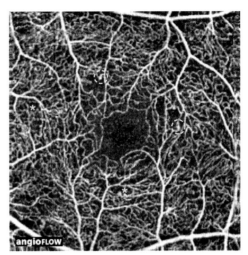

Fig. 15.7: Images obtained using the Angiovue optical coherence tomography angiography (OCTA) software of the RTVue XR Avanti (Optovue, Inc., Fremont, CA). 3 mm x 3 mm OCT angiogram of an eye with nonproliferative diabetic retinopathy (NPDR) showing an enlarged foveal avascular zone (FAZ), enlarged intercapillary spaces, a few microaneurysms (examples circled in yellow), and telangiectatic vessels (examples marked by yellow*).

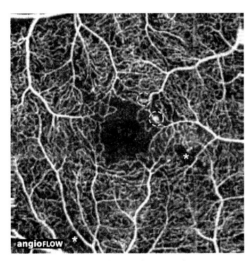

Fig. 15.8: Images obtained using the Angiovue optical coherence tomography angiography (OCTA) software of the RTVue XR Avanti (Optovue, Inc., Fremont, CA). 3 mm x 3 mm OCT angiogram of an eye with nonproliferative diabetic retinopathy (NPDR) showing an enlarged foveal avascular zone (FAZ), areas of capillary nonperfusion (examples marked by white *), and a few microaneurysms (examples circled in yellow).

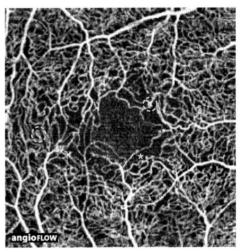

Fig. 15.9: Images obtained using the Angiovue optical coherence tomography angiography (OCTA) software of the RTVue XR Avanti (Optovue, Inc., Fremont, CA). 3 mm x 3 mm OCT angiogram of an eye with nonproliferative diabetic retinopathy (NPDR) showing an enlarged foveal avascular zone (FAZ), enlarged intercapillary spaces, a few microaneurysms (examples circled in yellow), and telangiectatic vessels (example marked by yellow *).

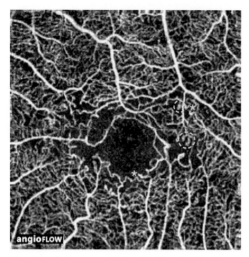

Fig. 15.10: Images obtained using the Angiovue optical coherence tomography angiography (OCTA) software of the RTVue XR Avanti (Optovue, Inc., Fremont, CA). 3 mm x 3 mm OCT angiogram of an eye with nonproliferative diabetic retinopathy (NPDR) showing a greatly enlarged foveal avascular zone (FAZ), surrounding microaneurysms (examples circled in yellow), and telangiectatic vessels (examples marked by yellow *).

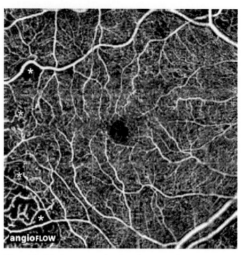

Fig. 15.11: Images obtained using the Angiovue optical coherence tomography angiography (OCTA) software of the RTVue XR Avanti (Optovue, Inc., Fremont, CA). 6 mm x 6 mm OCT angiogram of an eye with nonproliferative diabetic retinopathy (NPDR) showing large areas of capillary non-perfusion especially inferotemporally (examples marked by white *) and telangiectatic vessels (examples marked by yellow *).

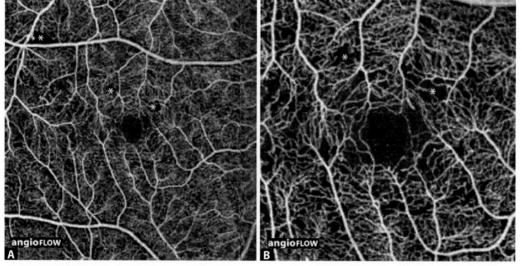

Figs 15.12A and B: Images obtained using the Angiovue optical coherence tomography angiography (OCTA) software of the RTVue XR Avanti (Optovue, Inc., Fremont, CA) of an eye with nonproliferative diabetic retinopathy (NPDR). (A) 6 mm x 6 mm OCT angiogram showing multiple areas of capillary nonperfusion (examples marked by white *). (B) 3 mm x 3 mm OCT angiogram to get better detail of the areas of capillary nonperfusion (examples marked by white *) and microaneurysms.

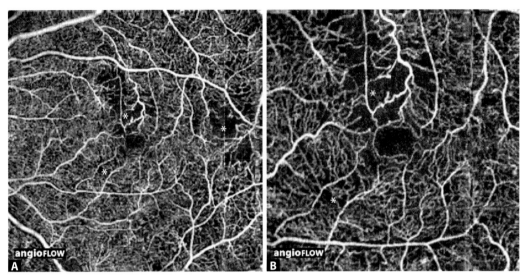

Figs 15.13A and B: Images obtained using the Angiovue optical coherence tomography angiography (OCTA) software of the RTVue XR Avanti (Optovue, Inc., Fremont, CA) of an eye with nonproliferative diabetic retinopathy (NPDR). (A) 6 mm x 6 mm OCT angiogram showing large areas of capillary nonperfusion (examples marked by white *), one of which is continuous with the foveal avascular zone (FAZ). (B) 3 mm x 3 mm OCT angiogram to get better detail of the drastic areas of capillary nonperfusion (examples marked by white *) and telangiectatic vessels.

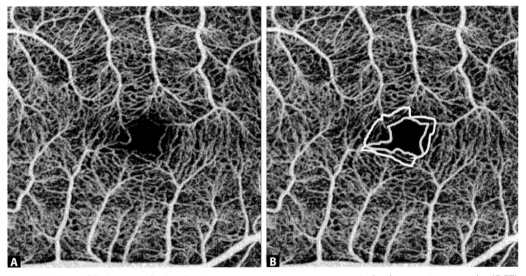

Figs 15.14A and B: Images obtained using a prototype swept source optical coherence tomography (OCT) system at 1,050 nm wavelength (Department of Electrical Engineering and Computer Science, Massachusetts Institute of Technology, Cambridge, MA). (A) 3 mm x 3 mm OCT angiogram of a nondiabetic eye. (B) The foveal avascular zone (FAZ) is demarcated in yellow and measures 0.16 mm^2 while the perifoveal intercapillary area is delineated in white and measures 0.35 mm^2.

can then be evaluated on the OCT angiogram to determine if neovascularization is present. Additionally, visualization of NVE and NVD is especially aided by segmentation to identify and project specific retinal layers. If the OCTA is segmented to create an OCT angiogram containing microvascular information between the RNFL and the top of the NVE, the abnormal vessels are much more easily appreciated (Fig. 15.21). A similar method can be employed in cases of NVD. As shown in Figure 15.22, the abnormal vessels can also be observed as tortuous vessels overlying the optic nerve, which is not observed in eyes without NVD.

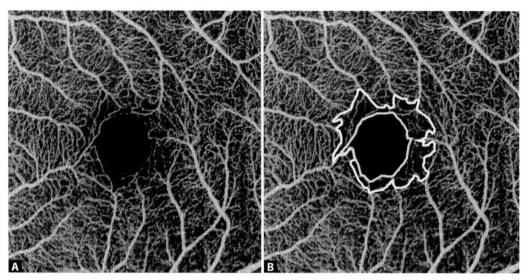

Figs 15.15A and B: Images obtained using a prototype swept source optical coherence tomography (OCT) system at 1,050 nm wavelength (Department of Electrical Engineering and Computer Science, Massachusetts Institute of Technology, Cambridge, MA). (A) 3 mm x 3 mm OCT angiogram of a diabetic eye without clinical retinopathy. The foveal avascular zone (FAZ) and perifoveal intercapillary area appear enlarged. (B) The FAZ is demarcated in yellow and measures 0.394 mm^2 while the perifoveal intercapillary area is delineated in white and measures 0.881 mm^2.

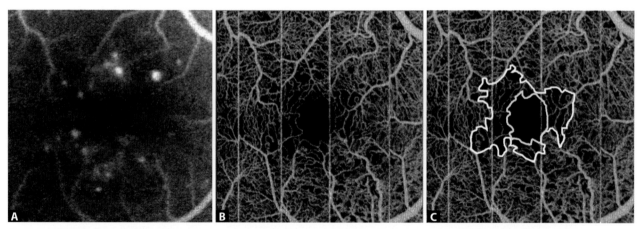

Figs 15.16A to C: Images obtained using a prototype swept source optical coherence tomography (OCT) system at 1,050 nm wavelength (Department of Electrical Engineering and Computer Science, Massachusetts Institute of Technology, Cambridge, MA). (A) Fluorescein angiography (FA) of an eye with nonproliferative diabetic retinopathy, which has been cropped to approximately a 3 mm x 3 mm area. It is not possible to exactly delineate the foveal avascular zone (FAZ) and perifoveal intercapillary area. (B) 3 mm x 3 mm OCT angiogram of the same eye. The FAZ and perifoveal intercapillary area appear enlarged. (C) The FAZ is demarcated in yellow and measures 0.314 mm^2 while the perifoveal intercapillary area is delineated in white and measures 1.125 mm^2.

SUMMARY

The major disadvantage of using OCTA in the diagnosis and management of diabetic retinopathy is the limited field of view since many clinically important changes occur in the periphery. Increasing the field of view results in lower *en face* image resolution. Various strategies have been employed to widen the field of view. This includes the montaging of multiple small field of view OCTA images to obtain a wider field of view. Some OCT instruments with motion tracking may be able to do this in an automated manner. In addition, future OCT technology will likely operate with higher A-scan acquisition speeds. This can

increase the field of view, however, it is important to note that in order to preserve *en face* image resolution, the number of A-scans will increase proportionally to the area, which is the square of the dimension. Therefore, significant increases in imaging speed are required.

In summary, OCTA is a powerful tool in the evaluation of diabetic retinopathy. It displays the retinal vasculature in great detail, allowing for identification of enlarged FAZ and perifoveal intercapillary area, subtle microvascular changes such as microaneurysms and areas of capillary nonperfusion, and neovascularization.

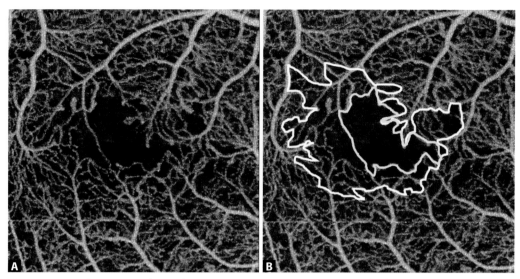

Figs 15.17A and B: Images obtained using a prototype swept source optical coherence tomography (OCT) system at 1,050 nm (Department of Electrical Engineering and Computer Science, Massachusetts Institute of Technology, Cambridge, MA). (A) 3 mm x 3 mm OCT angiogram of an eye with proliferative diabetic retinopathy. The foveal avascular zone (FAZ) and perifoveal intercapillary area appear greatly enlarged. (B) The FAZ is demarcated in yellow and measures 0.548 mm² while the perifoveal intercapillary area is delineated in white and measures 1.899 mm².

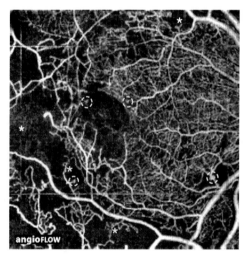

Fig. 15.18: Images obtained using the Angiovue optical coherence tomography angiography (OCTA) software of the RTVue XR Avanti (Optovue, Inc., Fremont, CA). 6 mm x 6 mm OCT angiogram of an eye with proliferative diabetic retinopathy (PDR) showing extreme areas of capillary non-perfusion (examples marked by white *), an enlarged foveal avascular zone (FAZ), telangiectatic vessels (examples marked by yellow *), and microaneurysm (examples circled in yellow).

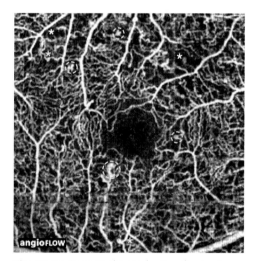

Fig. 15.19: Images obtained using the Angiovue optical coherence tomography angiography (OCTA) software of the RTVue XR Avanti (Optovue, Inc., Fremont, CA). 3 mm x 3 mm OCT angiogram of an eye with proliferative diabetic retinopathy (PDR) showing areas of capillary nonperfusion (examples marked by white *), telangiectatic vessels (examples marked by yellow *), and multiple microaneurysm throughout the macula (examples circled in yellow).

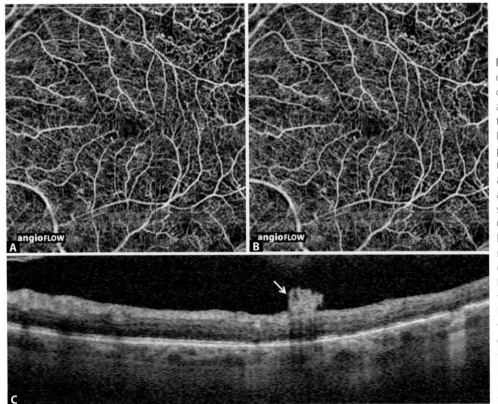

Figs 15.20A to C: Images obtained using the Angiovue optical coherence tomography angiography (OCTA) software of the RTVue XR Avanti (Optovue, Inc., Fremont, CA) of an eye with proliferative diabetic retinopathy (PDR). (A) 6 mm x 6 mm OCT angiogram of the inner retina with a green line showing the cross-section of the corresponding OCT B-scan shown in C and a red line indicating the location of the neovascularization elsewhere (NVE). (B) Same image as in (A) but without the lines blocking the view of the NVE. The NVE is difficult to differentiate from the surrounding vasculature. (C) Corresponding OCT B-scan from the cross-section of the green line in (A). The NVE (white arrow) is seen as tissue growing into the vitreous.

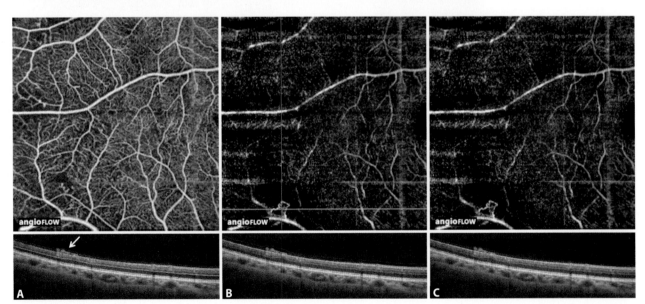

Figs 15.21A to C: Images obtained using the Angiovue optical coherence tomography angiography (OCTA) software of the RTVue XR Avanti (Optovue, Inc., Fremont, CA) of an eye with proliferative diabetic retinopathy (PDR). (A) 6 mm x 6 mm OCT angiogram and corresponding OCT B-scan of the inner retina. It is difficult to detect the neovascularization elsewhere (NVE) in the OCT angiogram. Abnormal tissue is seen growing into the vitreous on the OCT B-scan (white arrow). (B) 3 mm x 3 mm OCT angiogram segmented to show the section between the red and green lines as seen on the corresponding OCT B-scan. The horizontal green line on the OCT angiogram corresponds to the location of the OCT B-scan shown. The NVE is easily appreciable at the cross-section of the horizontal green and vertical red lines. (C) Same image as in (B) but without the lines blocking the view of the NVE on the OCT angiogram.

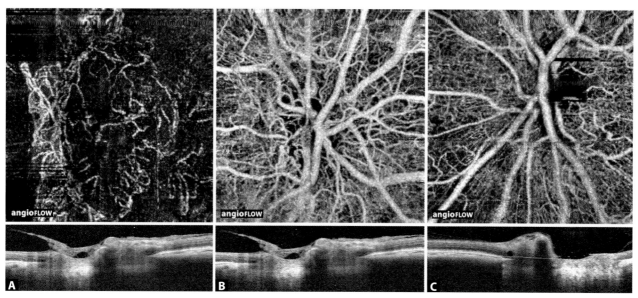

Figs 15.22A to C: Images obtained using the Angiovue optical coherence tomography angiography (OCTA) software of the RTVue XR Avanti (Optovue, Inc., Fremont, CA) of a patient with two eyes that have proliferative diabetic retinopathy (PDR). (A) 3 mm x 3 mm OCT angiogram of the patient's right eye segmented to show any vessels above the internal limiting membrane of the corresponding OCT B-scan. Neovascularization of the disc (NVD) is apparent. (B) The same 3 mm x 3 mm OCT angiogram in (A) segmented to show vessels between the internal limiting membrane (ILM) and Bruch's membrane. The tortuous NVD vessels arising from the optic disc can still be appreciated. (C) 3 mm x 3 mm OCT angiogram of the patient's left eye segmented in the same way as in (B). This eye does not have NVD. Other markers of diabetic retinopathy are shown such as telangiectatic vessels and areas of capillary nonperfusion.

OCT Angiography in Diabetic Retinopathy

André Romano, Rubens Belfort Jr

INTRODUCTION

Ophthalmic complications of hyperglycemia are most profound in cornea and retina. Retina accounts for the majority of visual loss in diabetics, and diabetic retinopathy is the most common cause of blindness in people over the age of 50. In addition, the diabetic choroid has vascular–related changes similar to those in the diabetic retina. Consequently, systematic evaluations of retinal and choroidal capillaries are essential.

Fluorescein angiography (FA) was introduced in the 60s as a method for visualizing the retinal and choroidal vessels and rapidly became the gold standard exam for identifying and classifying several of retinal vascular diseases.[1] The method is based on intravenous injection of a fluorescein dye to evaluate retinal vascular capillary network.

Leakage, capillary non-perfusion, vascular structural abnormalities, and neovascularization of the disc (NVD) and neovascularization elsewhere (NVE) are among the most common features observed in this technique in a patient with diabetic retinopathy. However, this technique is time-consuming, invasive and while considered harmless, the dyes pose risks ranging from nausea to allergic reactions, including anaphylaxis in rare instances death.

OPTICAL COHERENCE TOMOGRAPHY ANGIOGRAPHY TECHNIQUE

Optical coherence tomography angiography (OCTA) is a new non-invasive imaging technique that uses motion contrast imaging by comparing the decorrelation signal between sequential OCT B-scans acquired at the exact same cross-sectional image to generate a blood flow angiogram.[2]

Split-spectrum amplitude decorrelation angiography (SSADA) algorithm is the AngioVue software of the RTVue XR Avanti spectral-domain OCT (SD-OCT) (Optovue, Inc, Fremont, CA). It obtains volumetric scans of 304 × 304 A-scans at 70,000 A-scans per second in approximately 3.0 seconds.

Automated segmentation of superficial and deep inner retinal vascular plexuses, outer retina, and choriocapillaris can be observed in an automated software option of 2 × 2 mm, 3 × 3 mm, 6 × 6 mm, and 8 × 8 mm OCT angiograms.

OCTA in Diabetic Retinopathy

Diabetic retinopathy (DR) is a microvasculopathy that features: increased vascular permeability, microvasculature leaks and capillaries that are lost early in the disease. Hyperglycemia and mitochondrial and extracellular reactive oxygen species (ROS) are toxic to endothelial cells (ECs), pericytes, and neurons, resulting in their death early in DR. OCT angiography may help us to understand this pathophysiology in the course of the disease.

PRE-PROLIFERATIVE DIABETIC RETINOPATHY

The first changes observed at the pre-proliferative diabetic retinopathy patients imaged by OCT angiography are vascular remodeling bordering the foveal vascular zone (FAZ), followed by vascular tortuosity, narrowing of capillary lumens and dilation of its ends. These changes are best seen at the level of the superficial capillary plexus (Figs 16.1A to E).

Changes in the deep capillary plexus are more difficult to observe due to size and morphology of the capillaries but with the development of the disease these modifications may also be appreciated.

This mechanism is explained by endothelial cell death from hyperglycemia or leukocyte oxidative burst and subsequent increased vascular permeability appear to occur before pericyte

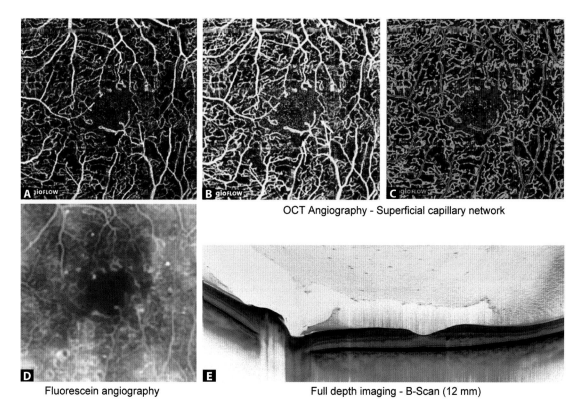

OCT Angiography - Superficial capillary network

Fluorescein angiography   Full depth imaging - B-Scan (12 mm)

Figs 16.1A to E: Non proliferative diabetic retinopathy: Optical coherence tomography angiography (OCTA) at the superficial vascular plexus (A to C) shows vascular remodeling bordering the foveal vascular zone (FAZ), capillary tortuosity, narrowing of capillary lumens and dilation of its terminals adjacent to FAZ. (D) These changes cannot be appreciated in the same manner in FA. (E) B-scan depicts discrete cystoid changes in the inner layer temporally to the fovea.

dropout occurs.[3] OCT-A has the disadvantage that it cannot visualize this vascular permeability, whereas FA shows dye leakage from abnormal retinal capillaries.

On the other hand, low perfusion is commonly seen when using a 3 x 3 mm OCT angiogram. (Figs 16.2A and B) Smaller size angiogram may also depict better vascular details than 6 x 6 mm or 8 x 8 mm (Figs 16.3A to C)

Visualization of microaneurysms is also well-delineated with smaller angiograms, but not all microaneurysms are observed in both superficial and deep capillary network, most probably because OCTA is limited by the principle of slowest detectable flow (Figs 16.4A to E).

Increased permeability of fluid and protein can result in diabetic macular edema (DME). Diabetic macular edema is the common cause of visual function loss in both nonproliferative and proliferative DR. These changes depict vascular loops in the presence of cysts in both superficial and deep vessels. En face OCT is the best technique to outline cystic changes in DME and inner plexiform layer appears to be the best location to appreciate fine details (Figs 16.5A to H).

Proliferation of retinal capillary endothelium initially causes intraretinal microvascular abnormalities (IRMA), small abnormal vascular formations in areas lacking viable capillaries.[4]

OCT angiography illustrates an IRMA at the superior temporal arcade along with reduced capillary density and adjacent non-

perfusion in a patient with severe non-proliferative diabetic retinopathy. Moreover, capillary shunts between superficial and deep capillary plexus can also be appreciated at this stage (Figs 16.6A and B)

Larger field of view allows better peripheral detection of microvascular changes, reduced capillary density and areas of capillary non-perfusion (Figs 16.7A to C).

PROLIFERATIVE DIABETIC RETINOPATHY

Endothelial cells proliferation and migration from veins and venules and chronic ischemia can result in the formation of preretinal neovascularization, the hallmark of proliferative retinopathy.

When new vessels are detected on the retina or the optic disc, diabetic retinopathy has progressed to the proliferative stage. In contrast to the abnormalities of nonproliferative retinopathy, those of proliferative retinopathy are no longer contained within the retina. Abnormal new blood vessels and connective tissue erupt through the surface of the retina or optic nerve to grow on the posterior surface of the vitreous (posterior hyaloid) or proliferate into the vitreous gel.

Modifying the *en face* OCT angiography slab toward the vitreous allows the operator to precisely evaluate, extend and

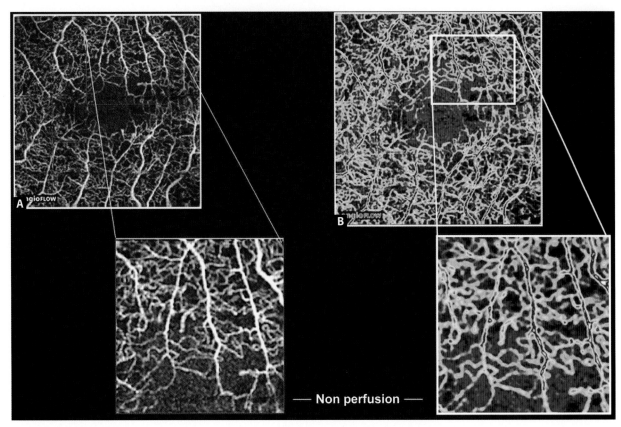

Figs 16.2A and B: Automated software option of smaller OCT angiograms demonstrates low perfusion (A-B). Modified two dimensional algorithm depicts superficial and deep superficial capillaries and area of low perfusion in one scan (B)

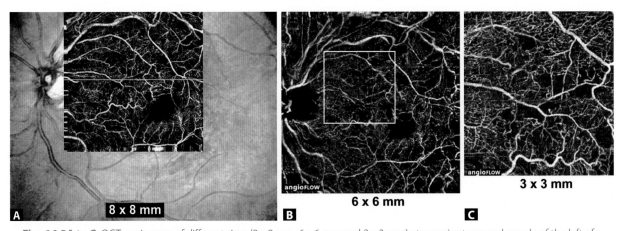

Figs 16.3A to C: OCT angiogram of different sizes (8 × 8 mm, 6 × 6 mm and 3 × 3 mm) at superior temporal arcade of the left of a patient with non-proliferative diabetic retinopathy (A-C). Note better vascular details and non-perfusion areas with 3 x 3 mm scan (C).

morphology of the network without the cumbersome of dye leakage. Large view angiograms such as 8 × 8 mm may help to locate neovascularization emanating from areas elsewhere in the retina (NVE) and along the temporal vascular arcades (Figs 16.8A to E).

OCTA has great potential for use in diabetic retinopathy because is noninvasive, provides accurate size and localization information, visualizes both superficial and deep capillary plexus but most important acquires volumetric scans that can be segmented to specific depths such as the vitreo-retinal interface to assess neovascularization.

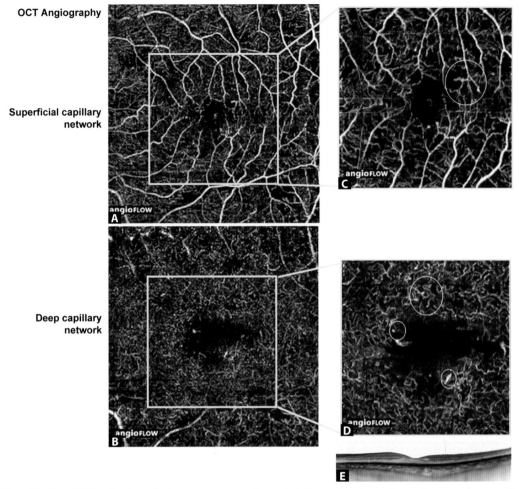

Figs 16.4A to E: Visualization of microaneurysms is also well-delineated with smaller angiograms, but not all microaneurysms is perceived in both superficial and deep capillary network, most probably because OCTA is limited by the principle of slowest detectable flow (A to D). (E) Cross section scan.

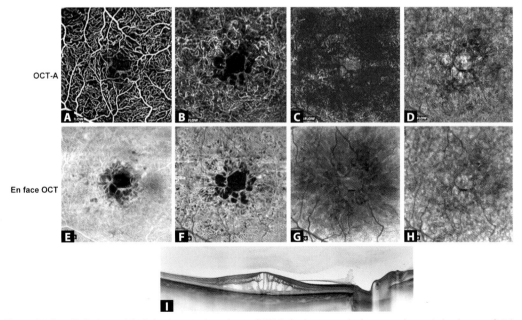

Figs 16.5A to H: Patient with diabetic macular edema. OCT-A depicts vascular loops and cysts in both superficial and deep plexus (A and B). *En face* OCT is best technique to outline cystic changes in DME and inner plexiform layer appears to be the best location to appreciate fine details (F). (I) Cross section scan.

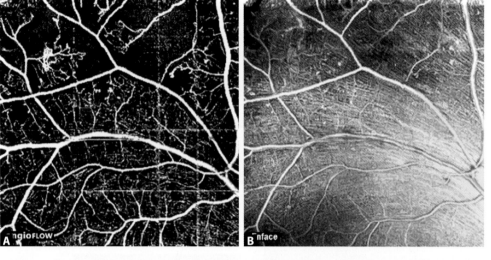

Figs 16.6A and B: OCT angiography illustrates an IRMA at the superior temporal arcade along with reduced capillary density and adjacent non-perfusion in a patient with severe non-proliferative diabetic retinopathy. Capillary shunts between superficial and deep capillary plexus can also be appreciated at this stage.

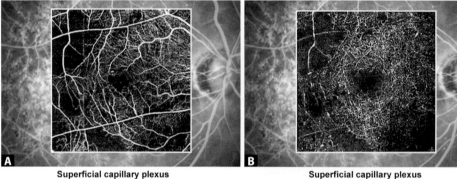

Superficial capillary plexus   Superficial capillary plexus

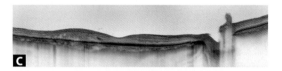

Figs 16.7A to C: Larger field of view (8 x 8 mm) allows better peripheral detection of microvascular changes, reduced capillary density and areas of capillary non-perfusion in both superficial and deep capillary plexus (A and B). (C) Cross section scan.

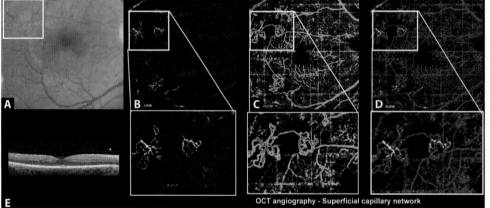

OCT angiography - Superficial capillary network

Figs 16.8A to E: Modifying the en face OCT angiography slab (E) toward the vitreous allows the operator to precisely evaluate, extend and morphology of the network without the cumbersome of dye leakage. Large view angiograms such as 8 x 8 mm may help to locate neovascularization emanating from areas elsewhere in the retina (NVE) and along the temporal vascular arcades (B to D).

REFERENCES

1. Novotny HR, Alvis DL. A method of photographing fluorescence in circulating blood in the human retina. Circulation. 1961;24:82–6.

2. Jia Y, Tan O, Tokayer J, Potsaid B, Wang Y, Liu JJ, Kraus MF, Subhash H, Fujimoto JG, Hornegger J, Huang D. Split-spectrum amplitude-decorrelation angiography with optical coherence tomography. Opt Express. 2012 Feb 13;20(4):4710-25. doi: 10.1364/OE.20.004710.

3. Tolentino MJ, Husain D, Theodosiadis P, et al. Angiography of fluid restricted anti-vascular endothelial growth factor antibody and dextrans in experimental choroidal neovascularization. Arch Ophthalmol. 2000;118:78–84.

4. Lutty GA, McLeod DS. A new technique for visualization of the human retinal vasculature. Arch Ophthalmol. 1992;110:267-76.

OCT Angiography Examination of Foveal Avascular Zone

Luca Di Antonio, Leonardo Mastropasqua

INTRODUCTION

Fifty years have passed since Novotny and Alvis have performed the first fluorescein angiography (FA). A simple, but invasive imaging method, that use intravenous fluorescein for producing and photographing fluorescence in circulating blood of the human retina.[1]

For many years, this revolutionary procedure has served as the gold standard method for imaging the retinal vasculature network and for estimating foveal avascular zone (FAZ) in many retinovascular disease.[2,3]

Foveal avascular zone is a capillary-free zone surrounded by interconnected retinal capillary beds. In agreement with anatomy, there is an absence of capillary network in the FAZ of approximately an average diameter of 500 to 600 micron.[4] The size of the FAZ reflects the condition of the microcapillary circulation in the foveal area and it is strongly positively correlated with the severity of capillary nonperfusion (dropout) in several retinovascular disease.[3]

The 'in vivo' quantification of FAZ shows potential for detecting and monitoring progression of vascular disease such as diabetic retinopathy, retinal vein occlusion, and macular teleangectasia. Previous study found that FAZ was significantly smaller in control eyes (median value 0.405 mm^2) than in eyes with background diabetic retinopathy (median value 0.737 mm^2) and in eyes with proliferative diabetic retinopathy (median value 0.866 mm^2) by means of FA.[5]

Optical coherence tomography angiography (OCTA) is a new dyeless method of imaging the retinal circulation providing a clean and continuous microvascular network around the FAZ[6,7] (Fig. 17.1).

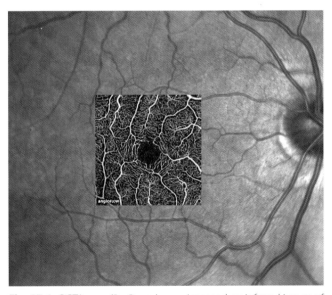

Fig. 17.1: OCTA scan (3 x 3 mm) superimposed on infrared image of 42-year-old man showing foveal avascular zone (FAZ) as a capillary-free zone surrounded by interconnected retinal capillary beds.

It allows to study separately the two vascular plexuses (superficial and deep) that have different features that cannot be distinguished by FA[7,8] (Fig. 17.2).

OCTA is an useful tool for assessing FAZ area in healthy (Fig. 17.3) and diseased subjects (Fig. 17.4).

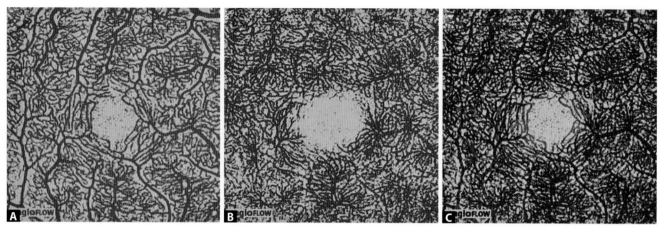

Figs 17.2A to C: Color-coded superficial vascular plexus (A) and deep vascular plexus (B) of a young healthy subject. Color-coded stack image showing superficial plexus made red and the deep plexus blue (C).

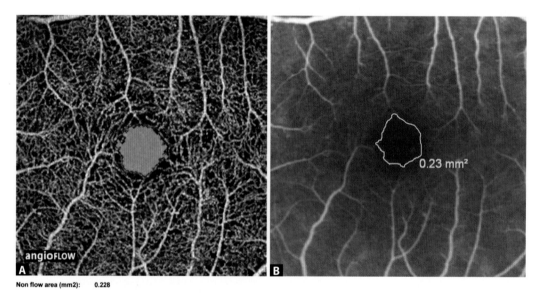

Non flow area (mm2):   0.228

Figs 17.3A and B: FAZ area estimated by OCT Angiography (A) and fluorescein angiography (B) in healthy subject. *Note* the same area in square millimeters measured in both noninvasive and invasive imaging techniques.

Vision-threatening retinovascular diseases such us diabetic retinopathy, retinal vein occlusion, and macular telangectasia involve retinal microcirculation by modifying the FAZ dimension (Figs 17.5 to 17.8). Capillary drop-out is positively correlated with FAZ enlargement (Fig. 17.7).

OCTA is able to detect the absence of FAZ in healthy[9] or diseased subjects affected by albinism[10] (Fig. 17.9).

These individuals show typical features of foveal hypoplasia. Capillaries can be seen to cross the central foveal area where capillaries are usually absent. This abnormal capillary patterns marked interindividual variation in capillary anatomy.[9] Then, we can observe a variation in shape and size of FAZ area in healthy subjects (Fig. 17.10).

In conclusion, OCTA provides noninvasive imaging of the retinal capillary network and FAZ in healthy and diseased eyes that is comparable, if not better, to invasive angiographic imaging.

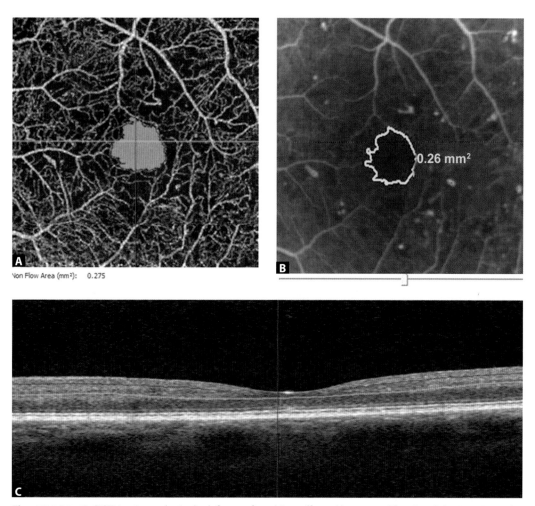

Von Flow Area (mm²): 0.275

Figs 17.4A to C: OCT Angiography in the left eye of a subject affected by nonproliferative diabetic retinopathy showing FAZ area measured as a 'no flow area' within the superficial vascular plexus (A). FAZ area measured by fluorescein angiography is indicated in square millimeters (B). Longitudinal OCT scan showing the reference plane of superficial vascular plexus (C).

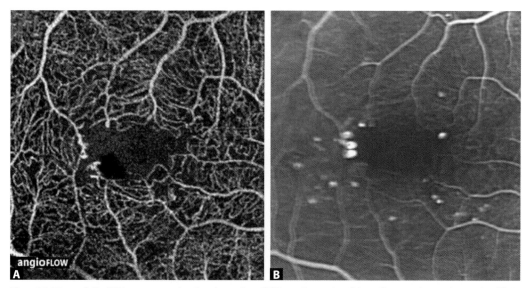

Figs 17.5A and B: FAZ area examination by using OCT angiography (A) or fluorescein angiography (B) in 79-year-old man with severe nonproliferative diabetic retinopathy showing typical features: Microaneurysms, capillary drop-out and FAZ enlargement.

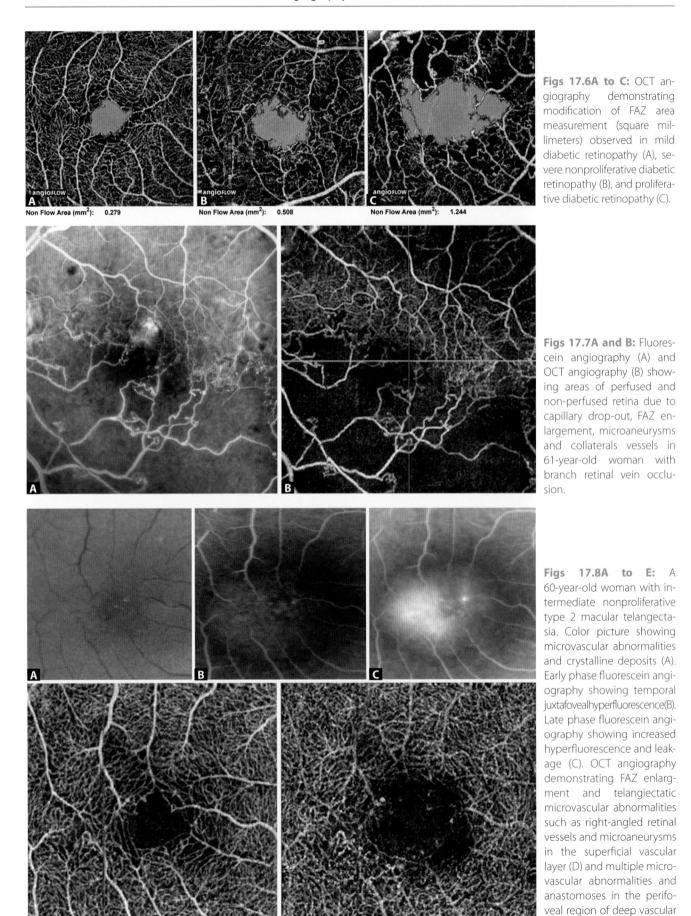

Figs 17.6A to C: OCT angiography demonstrating modification of FAZ area measurement (square millimeters) observed in mild diabetic retinopathy (A), severe nonproliferative diabetic retinopathy (B), and proliferative diabetic retinopathy (C).

Non Flow Area (mm^2):   0.279

Non Flow Area (mm^2):   0.508

Non Flow Area (mm^2):   1.244

Figs 17.7A and B: Fluorescein angiography (A) and OCT angiography (B) showing areas of perfused and non-perfused retina due to capillary drop-out, FAZ enlargement, microaneurysms and collaterals vessels in 61-year-old woman with branch retinal vein occlusion.

Figs 17.8A to E: A 60-year-old woman with intermediate nonproliferative type 2 macular telangectasia. Color picture showing microvascular abnormalities and crystalline deposits (A). Early phase fluorescein angiography showing temporal juxtafoveal hyperfluorescence(B). Late phase fluorescein angiography showing increased hyperfluorescence and leakage (C). OCT angiography demonstrating FAZ enlargment and telangiectatic microvascular abnormalities such as right-angled retinal vessels and microaneurysms in the superficial vascular layer (D) and multiple microvascular abnormalities and anastomoses in the perifoveal region of deep vascular layer (E).

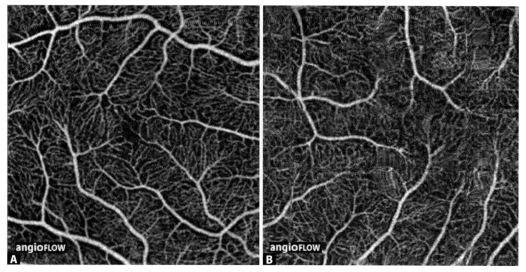

Figs 17.9A and B: OCT angiography of healthy young subject (A) and of child with albinism (B) detecting the absence of FAZ. *Note* retinal capillaries crossing the central foveal area where capillaries are usually absent.

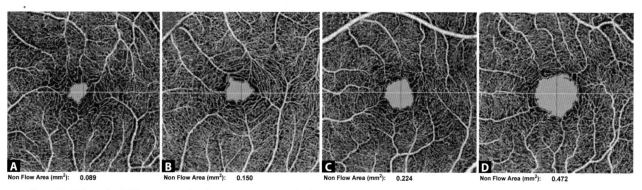

| Non Flow Area (mm²): 0.089 | Non Flow Area (mm²): 0.150 | Non Flow Area (mm²): 0.224 | Non Flow Area (mm²): 0.472 |

Figs 17.10A to D: OCT angiography showing interindividual variation in shape and size of FAZ area in young healthy subjects.

REFERENCES

1. Novotny HR, Alvis DL. A method of photographing fluorescence in circulating blood in the human retina. Circulation. 1961;24:82-6.

2. Laatikainen L. The fluorescein angiography revolution: a breakthrough with sustained impact. Acta Ophthalmol Scand. 2004;82:381-92.

3. Bresnick GH, Condit R, Syrjala S, et al. Abnormalities of the foveal avascular zone in diabetic retinopathy. Arch Ophthalmol. 1984;102:1286-93.

4. Zheng Y, Gandhi JS, Stangos AN. Automated segmentation of foveal avascular zone in fundus fluorescein angiography. Invest Ophthalmol Vis Sci. 2010;51:3653-9.

5. Mansour AM, Schachat A, Bodiford G, et al. Foveal avascular zone in diabetes mellitus. Retina. 1993;13:125-8.

6. Jia Y, Tan O, Tokayer J, et al. Split-spectrum amplitude decorrelation angiography with optical coherence tomography. Opt Express. 2012;20:4710-25.

7. Lumbroso B, Huang D, Jia Y, et al. Clinical Guide to Angio-OCT "Non Invasive Dyeless OCT Angiography. Jaypee Brothers Medical Publisher (P) Ltd. New Delhi, India, 2015.

8. Mastropasqua R, Di Antonio L, Di Staso S, et al. Optical coherence tomography angiography in retinal vascular diseases and choroidal neovascularization. J Ophthalmology. 2015;IN PRESS.

9. Sander B, Larsen M, Engler C, et al. Absence of foveal avascular zone demonstrated by laser scanning fluorescein angiography. Acta Ophthalmol (Copenh) 1994;72:550-2.

10. Mohammad S, Gottlob I, Kumar a, et al. The functional significance of foveal abnormalities in albinism measured using spectral-domain optical coherence tomography. Ophthalmology. 2011;118:1645-52.

OCT Angiography Examination in High Myopia

Luca Di Antonio, Leonardo Mastropasqua

Myopia is a complex disease affected by both environmental and genetic factors.[1]

The prevalence is lower in European, African and Pacific island individuals, and higher in Asian population (about 80%) where it seems to be attributed to reduction of the time that children spend outdoors.[1]

High myopia (HM) is a major cause of irreversible vision impairment.

Although the vision impairments associated with HM can be easily managed by therapeutic interventions, there is no intervention that can prevent the development and the progression of myopia.

By definition, HM is also known as degenerative or pathological myopia (PM). It refers to a condition in which individuals have an axial length >26 mm corresponding to a refractive error of at least –6.0 diopter.[2]

The anatomical basis of PM has been substantially enhanced by the application of imaging techniques, such as fluorescein angiography (FA), indocyanine green angiography (ICG-A), optical coherence tomography (OCT) and more recently by the introduction of OCT-angiography (OCT-A) into the daily clinical practice.[3]

The reasons for the development of myopic maculopathy are not clear, but it might simply be that excessive axial elongation thins the retina and choroid, and weakens the sclera.[4]

PM is accompanied by characteristic pathological changes including: Tessellated fundus (Fig. 18.1), temporal peripapillary atrophic crescent (Fig. 18.2), dome-shaped macula (Fig. 18.3), patchy atrophy (Fig. 18.4), lacquer cracks (Fig. 18.5), macular hemorrhages (Figs 18.5 and 18.6), and myopic choroidal neovascularization (mCNV) (Fig. 18.7). mCNV is the leading cause of vision loss in patients younger than 50 years and develops in 10% of highly myopic individuals.[5]

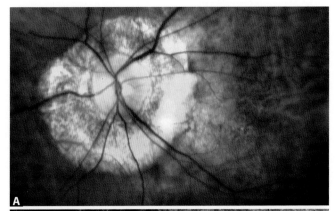
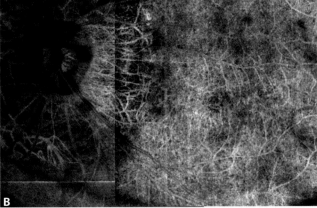

Figs 18.1A and B: (A) Color picture and (B) OCT-angiography showing typical tessellated fundus and peripapillary atrophy in a 48-year-old woman with pathological myopia.

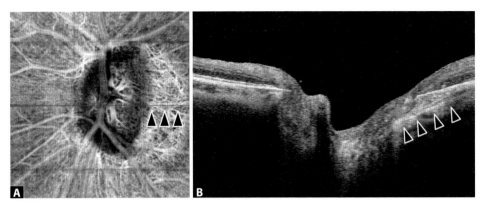

Figs 18.2A and B: (A) OCT-A and (B) longitudinal B scan showing temporal peripapillary atrophic crescent as an area of thin retina with enhancement of choroidal vessels (arrowheads) in a 55-year-old woman with high myopia.

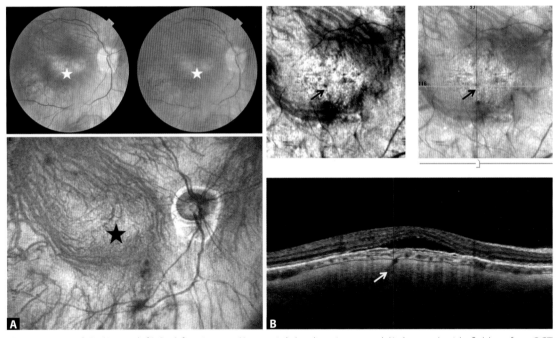

Figs 18.3A and B: (A, top left) Red free image, (A, top right) color picture and (A, bottom) wide field en-face OCT showing a dome shaped macula as a convex protrusion of the macula (star) within a new type of posterior pole staphyloma (bulge) in a 25-year-old man with high myopia. (B, top left) OCT-angiography, (B, top right) en-face OCT and (B, bottom) longitudinal OCT scan showing characteristic posterior bulge. *Note* short posterior ciliary arteries (arrow) perforating thickened sclera, and the presence of foveal detachment at the top of the dome-shaped macula.

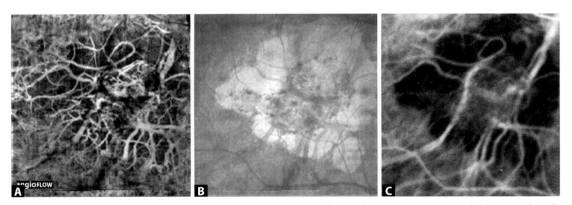

Figs 18.4A to C: Macular patchy atrophy in a 49-year-old woman with pathological myopia depicted as lesion with well-defined borders and enhanced choroidal vessels probably due to loss of choriocapillaris, degeneration of photoreceptor and the retinal pigment epithelium clearly visible in (A) OCT-angiography, (B) en-face OCT and (C) indocyanine green angiography images.

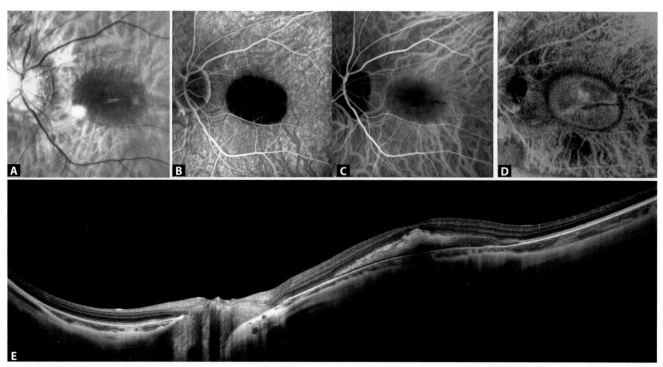

Figs 18.5A to E: (A) Color picture, (B and C) Fluorescein angiography and indocyanine green angiography late frames, (D) OCT-angiography and (E) widefield longitudinal B-scan showing macular hemorrhage above Bruch's membrane due to lacquer crack in a 31-year-old man with pathological myopia.

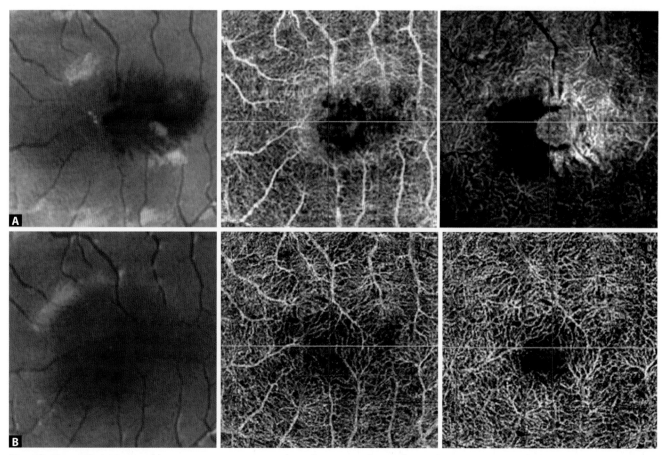

Figs 18.6A and B: A 29-year-old pregnant woman previously underwent to photorefractive keratectomy (PRK) for high myopia (-7diopters), (A, left) developed a macular hemorrhage visible in color picture (A, middle) involving superficial and (A, right) deep vascular plexuses. (B, left) Color picture of spontaneous resolution after one month (B, middle) with the restoration of both superficial and (B, right) deep vascular plexuses.

For many years, FA has served as the gold standard method for assessing the diagnosis and the treatment response to the antivascular endothelial growth factor (anti-VEGF) drugs[6] on the basis of late leakage observed in mCNV after dye injection.

OCT-A is a noninvasive tool, able to obtain flow imaging of retinal and choroidal microcirculation using the normal movement of the red blood cells into capillaries as intrinsic contrast medium.[3,7]

OCT-A enhances mCMV as an irregular or glomerular flow formation of new choroidal vessels surrounded by a hemorrhage (Fig. 18.7) or thin capsule (Fig. 18.8A). It is useful for the follow-up in patients treated with intravitreal injection of anti-VEGF showing a partial regression of the neovascular network (Figs 18.8 and 18.9) and enlargement of the patchy atrophy (Fig. 18.9B).

Sometimes in correspondence of patchy atrophy areas can be highlighted peculiar scleral changes of PM eyes, characterized by focal ectasia (Fig. 18.10).[8]

The combination of vitreous tractions forces with posterior staphyloma (Fig. 18.11), leads to vitreo-retinal disorders such as myopic retinoschisis with macular hole (Fig. 18.12),[9] and

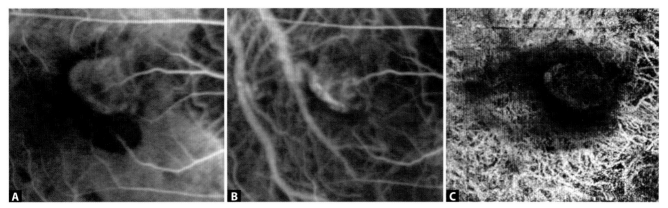

Figs 18.7A to C: (A) Fluorescein angiography, (B) green indocyanine angiography and (C) color-coded OCT-angiography showing myopic CNV surrounded by intraretinal hemorrhage. The new vessels are more enhanced with OCT-angiography image than fluorescein or indocyanine angiograms that produce immediate masking effect due to dye leakage.

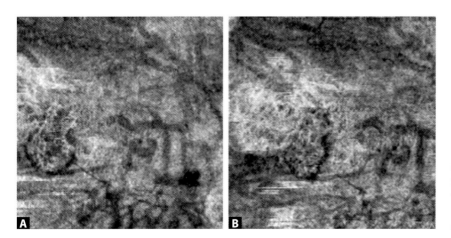

Figs 18.8A and B: (A) OCT-angiography showing myopic choroidal neovascularization surrounded by a thin capsule in a 34-year-old woman. (B) *Note* the partially regression of the new-vessels 24 hours after intravitreal injection of anti-VEGF.

peripapillary detachment (Fig. 18.13).[10] Then highly myopic eyes have a higher incidence of retinal detachment (Fig. 18.14) resulting from breaks in the peripheral retina.

In conclusion, OCT-A provides noninvasive imaging of the retinal and choroidal changes in PM that are comparable, if not better, to invasive angiographic imaging.

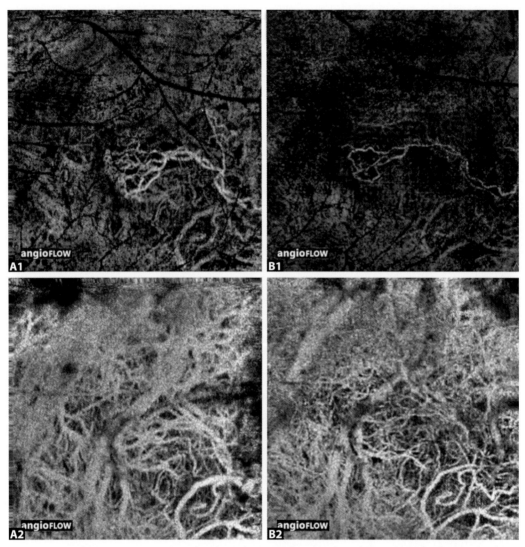

Figs 18.9A and B: OCT-angiography scan adapted to RPE reference plane showing (A1) feeder vessels of thin glomerular choroidal neovascularization of a 56-year-old at baseline (A2) in correspondence of a patchy atrophy area clearly visible in the scan adapted to choroid. (B1) Regression of the neovascularization after anti-VEGF intravitreal injection. (B2) *Note* the enlargement of the patchy atrophy area and a narrowing of the choroidal vessels caliber probably due to the ischemic effect of the anti-VEGF drugs.

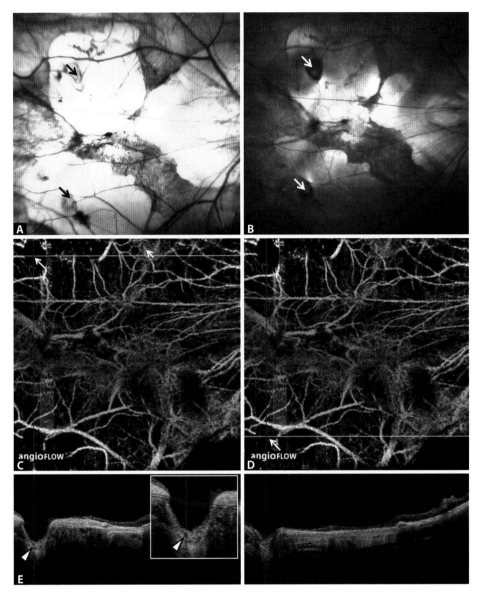

Figs 18.10A to E: (A) Color picture (B) infrared image (C-D) OCT-angiography and (E and F) longitudinal B scans of a 67-year-old man with pathological myopia showing scleral focal ectasia as two deep, dark oval lesions with well-defined borders (arrows) surrounded by patchy atrophy crossed by vessels. *Note* the vessel (arrowhead) perforating sclera at the bottom of the ectasia (E, enlarged view, arrowhead).

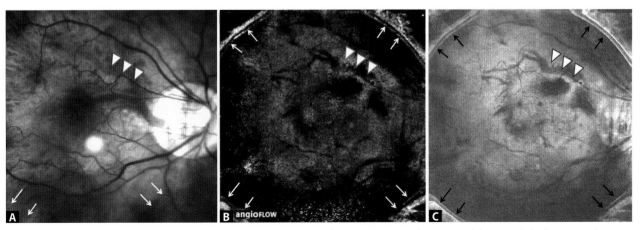

Figs 18.11A to C: (A) Color picture, (B) OCT-angiography, and (C) en-face OCT images of a 45-year-old man with high myopia showing posterior staphyloma borders (arrows) and large choroidal vessels (arrowheads).

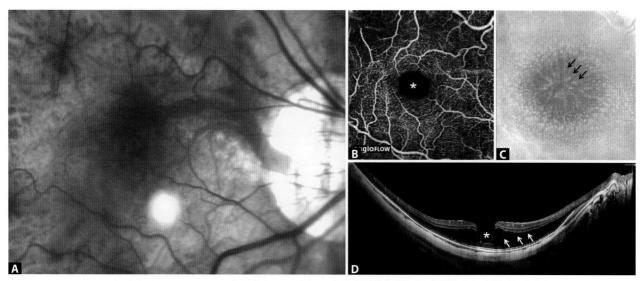

Figs 18.12A to D: (A) Color picture, (B) OCT-angiography, (C) en-face OCT, and (D) longitudinal B scan images of a 45-year-old man showing myopic retinoschisis with radial stretching of Müller cells pillars (arrows) and lamellar macular hole (*).

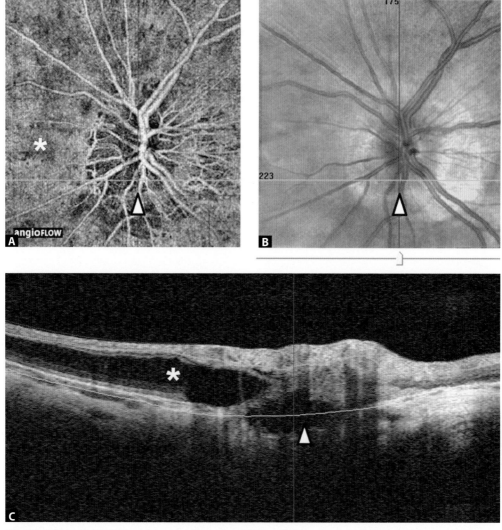

Figs 18.13A to C: (A) OCT-angiography, (B) en-face OCT and (C) longitudinal B scan of a 31-year-old woman showing peripapillary detachment in pathological myopia with retinoschisis (*) and intrachoroidal cavitation (arrowhead).

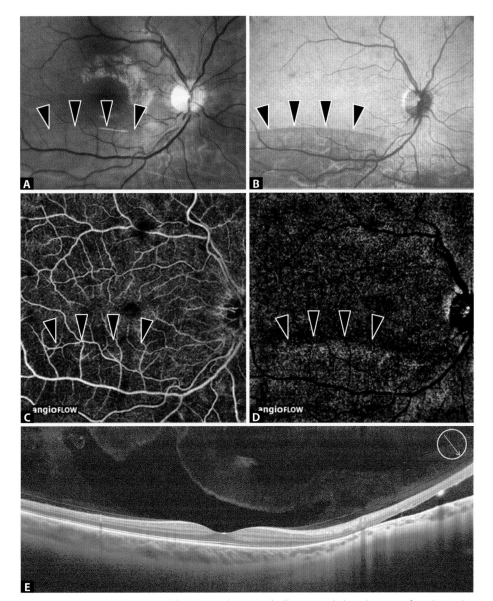

Figs 18.14A to E: A 25-year-old woman showing shallow retinal detachment inferiorly to the macula due to peripheral retinal break. (A) Color picture, (B) wide field *en face* OCT projection, (C) OCT-angiography scans in correspondence of the superficial vascular plexus and (D) outer retina (D) showing demarcation of subretinal fluid that laps perifoveal zone (arrowheads). (E) Widefield enhanced longitudinal B-scan demonstrating premacular bursa, incomplete posterior vitreous detachment with vitreomacular adhesion and the presence of subretinal fluid.

REFERENCES

1. Rose KA, Morgan IG, Ip J, et al. Outdoor activity reduces the prevalence of myopia in children. Ophthalmology. 2008;115:1279-85.
2. Curtin B, Karlin D. Axial length measurements and fundus changes of the myopic eye. Am J Ophthalmol. 1971;71:42-53.
3. Lumbroso B, Huang D, Jia Y, et al. Clinical Guide to Angio-OCT (NonInvasive, Dyeless OCT Angiography) Jaypee-Highlights medical publishers, Inc. 2014.
4. Morgan IG, Matsui KO, Saw SM. Myopia. Lancet. 2012;379:1739-48.
5. Ohno-Matsui K, Yoshida T, Futagami S, et al. Patchy atrophy and lacquer cracks predispose to the development of choroidal neovascularisation in pathological myopia. Br J Ophthalmol. 2003;87:570-73.
6. Cohen SY. Anti-VEGF drugs as the 2009 first-line therapy for choroidal neovascularization in pathologic myopia. Retina. 2009;29:1062-66.
7. Mastropasqua R, Di Antonio L, Di Staso S, et al. Optical coherence tomography angiography in retinal vascular diseases and choroidal neovascularization. Journal of Ophthalmology. 2015 IN PRESS.
8. Pedinielli A, Souied EH, Perrenoud F, et al. In vivo visualization of perforating vessels and focal scleral ectasia in pathological myopia. Invest Ophthalmol Vis Sci. 2013;54:7637-43.
9. Panozzo G, Mercanti A. Optical coherence tomography findings in myopic traction maculopathy. Arch Ophthalmol. 2004;122:1455-60.
10. Toranzo J, Cohen SY, Erginary A, et al. Peripapillary intrachoroidal cavitation in myopia. Am J Ophthalmol. 2005;140:731-2.

OCT Angiography Examination of Choroidal Nevi and Melanomas

Gilda Cennamo

PIGMENTED CHOROIDAL LESIONS

The relative differentiation between small choroidal melanoma and nevus can be challenging (Figs 19.1 and 19.2).

The criteria predicting the behavioral pattern of pigmented choroidal lesions have been developed by Shields et al: The thickness of the lesion; the presence of subretinal fluid; orange pigment in the lesion; the distance from the margins to the optic disc of <3 mm; change in the reflectivity at ultrasound examination and an absence of drusen, are used for early detection of small melanomas.[1,2]

Fourier domain optical coherence tomography (FD-OCT) provides structural information about the effects of choroidal nevus and melanoma on the retinal morphology but not about vascular tissue.

Optical coherence tomography angiography (Angio-OCT) is a new functional OCT based on high-resolution imaging techniques whereby the retinal and choroidal circulation may be visualized without the need of injecting any contrast agent.[3] It is now possible to use this new technique for the diagnosis and follow-up of choroidal nevi and small melanomas, as it visualizes the vascular tissue inside the tumor.

Choroidal Nevi

Angio-OCT imaging of choroidal nevi does not show a blood flow inside the outer nuclear layer (ONL), and the choroid capillary layer is normal.

Choroidal Melanomas

On the contrary, angio-OCT imaging of choroidal melanomas shows a dense irregular and fragmented vascular network inside the ONL and choroid capillary layers. In fact, coarse networks with blood flow are visible, which form an irregular spiderweb inside the tumor.

Moreover, angiochoroid capillary shows a hyporeflective area surrounded by a hyperreflective edged ring due to vascular tissue, in direct relation to the melanoma.

In conclusion, angio-OCT of choroidal nevi and melanomas may be used to visualize the tumor area, and is a viable non-invasive technique alongside echographic examination in the diagnosis of this pathology. Furthermore, it may be used to detect minimal morphological changes during follow-up of the choroidal nevi and after treatment of small choroidal melanomas (Fig. 19.3 to 19.5).

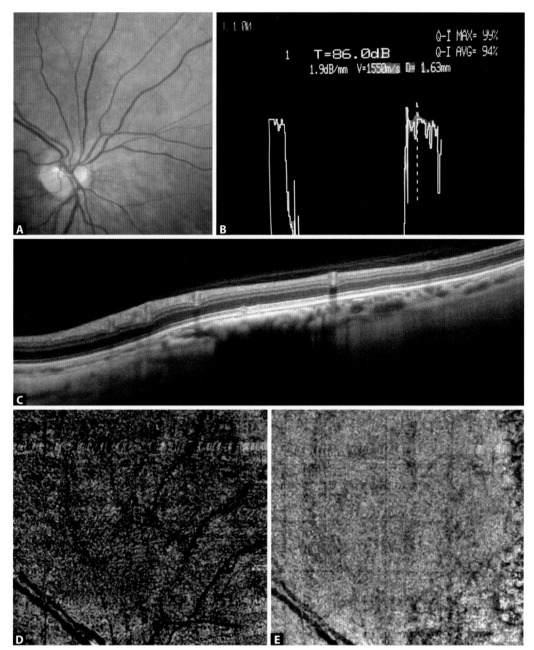

Figs 19.1A to E: Choroidal nevus. (A) Color fundus image showing a flat and well-demarcated melanocytic nevus. (B) A standardized echographic scan showing high reflectivity with irregular structures of the lesion. (C) Fourier domain optical coherence tomography. The lesion is distinguished from the surrounding normal choroid as highly reflective band with posterior shadowing. (D) Angio-outer retina does not show a blood flow inside the ONL. (E) Angio-choroid capillary shows normal vascular structure.

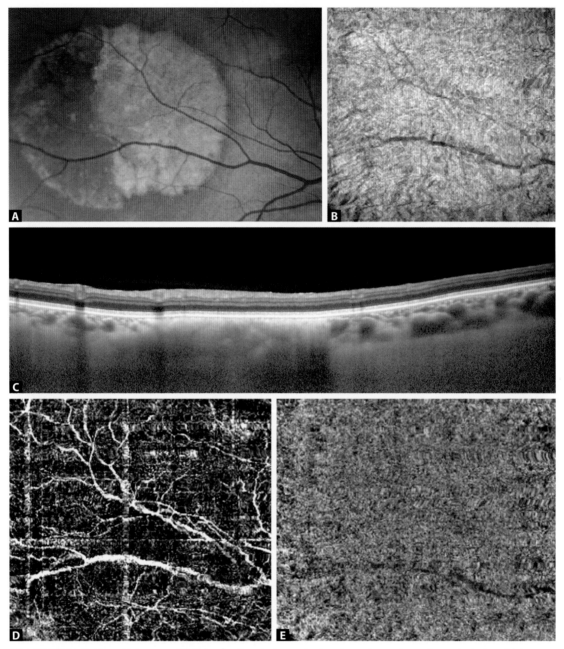

Figs 19.2A to E: Choroidal nevus. (A) Color fundus photograph showing a hyper-hypopigmented choroidal nevus. (B) *En face* optical coherence tomography showing a slight hyperreflective lesion. (C) Fourier domain optical coherence tomography reveals a sharply highly reflective band at the Bruch's/retinal pigment epithelium/choriocapillaris layer and posterior shadowing. (D and E) Angio-outer retina and angiochoroid capillary show normal vascular structure.

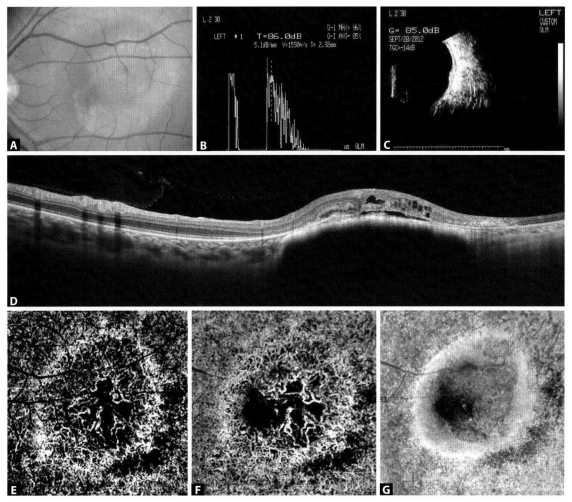

Figs 19.3 A to G: Choroidal melanoma. (A) Color fundus photograph showing a mildly elevated and pigmented choroidal lesion. (B) An A scan standardized echography shows a medium-low reflectivity of the lesion. (C) B scan ultrasound shows a slightly irregular dome-shaped mass (D) Fourier domain optical coherence tomography shows elevation of the retina-choroid with intra- and subretinal fluid. (D and E) Angio-outer retina and angiochoroid capillary reveal irregular vascular network inside the lesion. (F) *En face* optical coherence tomography shows a hyporeflective area with an irregular and hyperreflective edged ring.

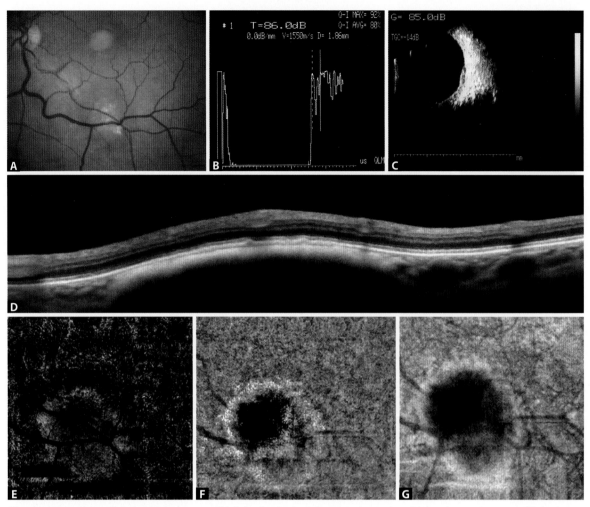

Figs 19.4A to G: Small choroidal melanoma. (A) Color fundus imaging showing a choroidal melanocytic tumor. (B) An A scan standardized echography shows a medium-low reflectivity of the lesion. B scan ultrasound shows a slight dome-shaped mass. (C) Fourier domain optical coherence tomography reveals the dome-shaped elevation of the choroid. (D to F) Angio-outer retina, angio-choroid capillary and *En face* optical coherence tomography show a hypo-hyperreflective irregular area due to vascular tissue.

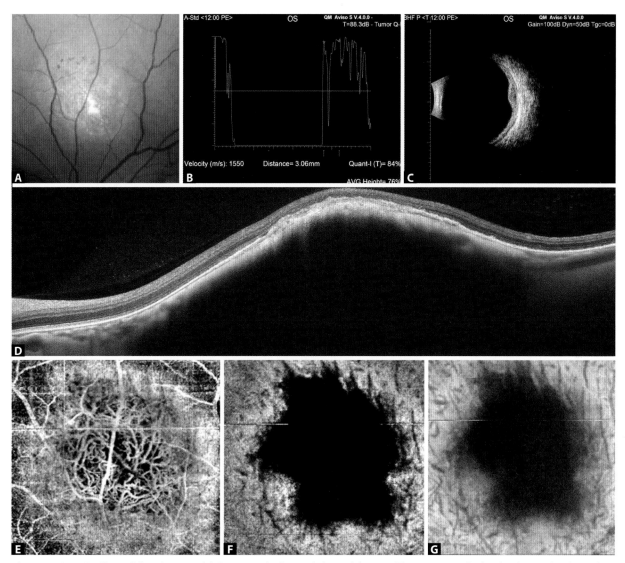

Figs 19.5A to G: Choroidal melanoma. (A) Pigmented, elevated choroidal mass; (B) A scan standardized echography shows low internal reflectivity of the lesion. (C) B-scan ultrasound shows a hyper reflective dome-shaped mass; (D) Fourier domain optical coherence tomography shows a middle elevation of choroid/retina complex, overlying the dome-shaped elevation of the choroid is a thickened irregular RPE; (E) Angio-outer retina reveals blood flow inside the tumor; (F and G) Angiochoroid capillary and *En face* optical coherence tomography shows a hyporeflective area with irregular and hyperreflective edged ring.

REFERENCES

1. Shields CL, Materin MA, Shields JA. Review of optical coherence tomography for intraocular tumors. Curr Opin Ophthalmol. 2005;16(3):141-54.

2. Shah SU, Kaliki S, Shields CL, et al. Enhanced depth imaging optical coherence tomography of choroidal nevus in 104 cases. Ophthalmology. 2012;119(5):1066-72.

4. Lumbroso B, Rispoli M, Savastano MC et al. Clinical Applications: Aspects of OCT SSADA angiography in eye desorders. In: Lumbroso B, Huang D (Eds). Clinical Guide for Angio-OCT. New Delhi, IN: Jaypee Brothers Medical Pub. 2015;pp.23-59.

OCT Angiography Examination in Glaucoma

David Huang, Michel Puech, Yali Jia, Simon S Gao, Liang Liu

INTRODUCTION

Glaucoma is associated with reduced blood flow in the optic nerve head (ONH) and retina. But up until now, there has been no practical method to measure this in the clinic. Optical coherence tomography (OCT) angiography of ONH blood flow using a swept-source OCT system has been found to be an accurate method to detect glaucoma.[1] Furthermore, the ONH flow index was highly correlated with visual field indices. The commercially available RTVue-XR Avanti (Optovue, Inc.) is a high-speed (70 kHz) 840 nm spectral OCT system that is able to map a large area of peripapillary retinal blood flow, which is also highly correlated with glaucoma status and the severity of visual field damage. Thus, OCT angiography of the ONH and peripapillary retina may add valuable new information for glaucoma assessment that complement conventional structural OCT measurements of the peripapillary retinal nerve fiber layer (NFL) thickness and macular ganglion cell complex or ganglion cell layer thickness.

QUANTIFICATION OF PERIPAPILLARY RETINAL FLOW INDEX AND VESSEL DENSITY

The examples in this chapter were obtained with the Avanti OCT system. In the *en face* OCT angiogram of the normal eye (Figs 20.1A and B), the peripapillary retina shows a dense microvascular network. In comparison, the glaucomatous eye shows reduced density of the peripapillary microvascular network (Figs 20.1E and F) with patches of nonperfusion that correlated well with the locations of NFL and visual field (VF) defects. Inside the ONH, both the normal and glaucomatous eyes showed areas of nonperfusion. The loss of both flow and reflectance signal in the

normal ONH are located in the large retinal vessels and is most likely due to the interferometric fringe washout associated with high velocity flow. Spectral OCT is more susceptible to the fringe washout effect (Figs 20.1C to H).[2] As a result, flow index and vessel density measurements inside the optic nerve heard (ONH) were unreliable. Since this artifact did not interfere with spectral OCT angiography outside the ONH, accurate quantification of peripapillary retinal perfusion is still possible and is the preferred method of glaucoma evaluation using spectral OCT.

To quantify the peripapillary retinal blood flow, the anatomic boundaries are first established. The disk boundary was drawn along the neural canal opening using structural OCT images. The peripapillary region was defined to be a 0.7 mm wide elliptical annulus extending outward from the optic disc boundary (Figs. 20.1B, F, between green circles). The peripapillary retinal flow index was defined as the average decorrelation value on the *en face* retinal angiogram in the peripapillary region. The vessel density was defined as the percentage area occupied by blood vessels in the peripapillary region in the *en face* retinal OCT angiogram. The peripapillary flow index and vessel density in the normal eye were 0.086 and 88.5%, respectively. The peripapillary flow index and vessel density in the glaucoma eye were lower at 0.070 and 78.9%, respectively.

CORRELATION BETWEEN PERIPAPILLARY RETINAL OCT ANGIOGRAM, NERVE FIBER MAP, AND VISUAL FIELD

Peripapillary retinal nonperfusions are associated with areas of NFL thinning, ganglion complex thinning, and VF defects (Fig. 20.2). These diagnostic modalities are synergistic.

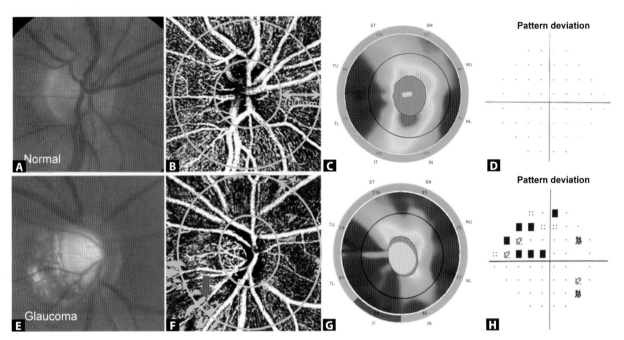

Figs 20.1A to H: Examples of a normal (top row) and glaucomatous (bottom row) right eye. Disc photographs (A, E), *en face* OCT angiograms of optic disc and peripapillary retina (3×3 mm)(B, F), retinal nerve fiber layer (NFL) thickness maps with octant classifications (C, G), and visual field (VF) pattern deviation maps (D, H) in a representative normal eye (top row) and perimetric glaucoma eye (bottom row). Nonperfusion areas in the peripapillary retina were highlighted in blue on the OCT angiograms. An inferotemporal arcuate nonperfusion area (purple arrow, F) in the glaucomatous angiogram correlated well with the NFL defect (G) and superior arcuate VF defect (H). Areas of flow voids (black) can be seen in the large retinal vessels inside the optic discs of both the normal (B) and glaucomatous (F) eyes. These are caused by interferometric fringe washout associated with high flow velocity.

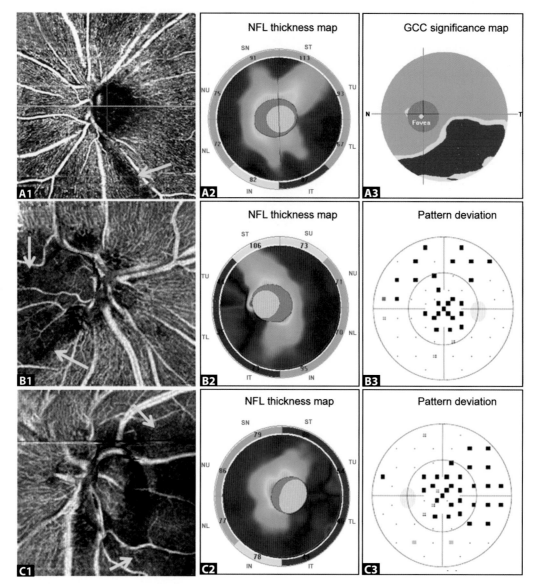

Figs 20.2A to C: Three eyes of 2 glaucoma patients separated into rows. *En face* OCT angiograms of the optic disc and peripapillary retina (left column), retinal nerve fiber layer (NFL) thickness maps with octant classifications (middle column), ganglion cell complex (GCC) significance map (right column A3), and visual field (VF) pattern deviation maps (left column B2, C3). (A) An inferotemporal arcuate nonperfusion area (yellow arrow, A1) on the *en face* angiogram correlated well with the inferotemporal NFL loss (red octant, A2) and inferior arcuate GCC defect (A3). (B) Right and (C) left eyes of a patient with broad areas of temporal nonperfusion on the OCT angiogram (between yellow arrows, B1, C1) that correlated well with temporal NFL loss (B2, C2) and central, superior, and nasal scotomas (B3, C3).

REFERENCES

1. Jia Y, et al. Quantitative OCT angiography of optic nerve head blood flow. Biomed Opt Express. 2012;3:3127-37, doi:10.1364/BOE.3.003127173662 [pii].

2. Hendargo HC, McNabb RP, Dhalla AH, Shepherd N, Izatt JA. Doppler velocity detection limitations in spectrometer-based versus swept-source optical coherence tomography. Biomed Opt Express. 2011;2:2175-88, doi:10.1364/BOE.2.002175148231 [pii].

PART 3

Future Developments in
OCT Angiography

Section Outline

Ultrahigh Speed Swept Source Technology for OCT Angiography

Eric M Moult, WooJhon Choi, Nadia K Waheed,
Talisa de Carlo, Jay S Duker, James G Fujimoto

This chapter presents an overview of future OCT technology for OCT angiography (OCTA), with a focus on ultrahigh speed, swept source OCT (SS-OCT). While the technology described herein is not yet commercially available, the results presented underscore the potential of OCTA as the next generation of technology becomes available in ophthalmology. Imaging speed is especially important for OCTA because OCTA protocols require repeated scanning of the same fundus position. In addition, OCTA is typically displayed *en face*, and therefore each pixel in the image requires multiple A-scans. For this reason, *en face* OCTA requires significant trade-offs between image acquisition time, retinal coverage, and *en face* pixel resolution. Ultrahigh speed imaging systems are critical to improving retinal coverage and pixel resolution while still maintaining clinically practical imaging times.

SS-OCT FOR ULTRAHIGH SPEED

The most promising approach for achieving ultrahigh speed is a technique known as swept source/Fourier domain OCT. Swept source OCT (SS-OCT) uses an interferometer with a frequency swept, narrow line width laser, rather than a broadband light source, spectrometer, and line scan camera, which are used in spectral domain OCT (SD-OCT).[1,2] SS-OCT can achieve much faster imaging speeds than SD-OCT because the speeds are not limited by camera reading rates. In addition, SS-OCT enables imaging with longer, ~1,050 nm, wavelength light, a wavelength at which conventional line scan cameras have limited sensitivity. OCT at 1,050 nm wavelengths suffers less scattering loss from cataracts and ocular opacities, and tissue image penetration is improved compared to the 850 nm wavelengths typically used in SD-OCT instruments.[3,4] Combined, these advantages enable SS-OCT to achieve ultrahigh speeds as well as better imaging of structures such as the choroid and choriocapillaris.

How SS-OCT Works

Figure 21.1 shows a schematic of how swept source/Fourier domain detection works. Swept source/Fourier domain detection uses a narrow bandwidth, frequency swept light source with an interferometer. The interference output is detected with a high speed photodetector, without the need for a spectrometer and line scan camera. In swept source/Fourier domain detection, different echo time delays of light are encoded as different oscillation frequencies when the laser light source is frequency swept. The echo time delays can be measured by Fourier transforming the detector signal to extract the oscillation frequencies. Swept source/Fourier domain detection can also be understood by noting that the light source frequency sweep essentially labels different times with different frequencies. The output from the swept light source is split into two paths. One light path is directed onto tissue and light is backreflected or backscattered from tissue structures at different depths. The other path is reflected from a fixed (i.e. not scanned) reference mirror at a given delay. The light from the tissue and the reference have a relative time delay Δz related to the depth of the tissue structure. The interference of the signal and reference light will produce an oscillation or beat frequency because there is a frequency difference between the two light waves at the detector. The oscillation frequency will be related to the echo time delay Δz. Larger echo delays will produce higher frequency oscillations. Similar to spectral/Fourier domain detection, the echo delays or A-scans can be measured by Fourier transforming the detector signal acquired over one frequency sweep of the light source. Each frequency sweep of the light source generates one A-scan and the A-scan imaging rate is determined by the sweep repetition rate of the light source.

Swept source techniques were used 20 years ago for fiber-optics/photonics measurement as well as laser radar. SS-OCT

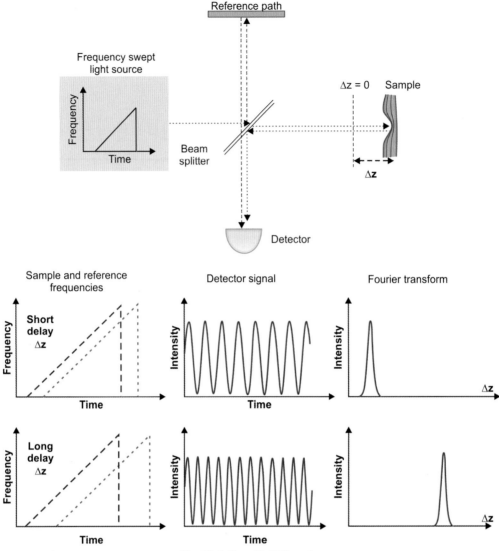

Fig. 21.1: How SS-OCT works.

was demonstrated by our group as early as 1997 by Chinn et al.[2] and Golubovic et al.,[1] but performance was limited by available laser technology. Increases in SS-OCT imaging speed have been closely linked to advances in lasers, because A-scan rates are determined by the laser sweep repetition rate. In 2003, Yun et al. demonstrated OCT imaging with 19,000 A-scans per second and 13–14 um axial resolution (in air).[5] Imaging speeds of 115,000 A-scans per second were achieved using swept laser technology with a diffraction grating and rotating polygon mirror tuner in 2005.[6] The development of a new swept laser technology known as Fourier domain mode locking or FDML (not related to Fourier domain OCT) by Huber et al. in 2006 overcame fundamental limitations to laser sweep speed and enabled dramatic increases in imaging speed.[7] In 2008, Srinivasan et al. used FDML lasers to demonstrate retinal imaging at 249,000 A-scans per second and 1050 nm wavelength with an 8 μm axial resolution.[8] Ultrahigh speed retinal imaging at 1,370,000 A-scans per second was demonstrated by Klein et al. in 2011 using FDML lasers, but these extremely high speeds required performance tradeoffs; image resolution was 19 um and sensitivity was 92 dB.[9]

The availability and cost of swept laser technology is the major limiting factor for commercializing next generation SS-OCT. Commercially available swept lasers at 1,050 nm using polygon mirror swept filter technology were employed for swept source OCT retinal imaging at 28,000 A-scans per second and 10 um axial resolution as early as 2007.[10] Commercial swept lasers using short cavities and microelectromechanical systems (MEMS) tunable filter technology could achieve higher imaging speeds of 100,000 to 200,000 A-scans per second with 7 um axial resolution.[11] The most recent advances have been achieved by vertical cavity surface emitting (VCSEL) swept laser technology. Imaging speeds of 580,000 A-scans per second were recently demonstrated at 1,050 nm with 9 um axial resolution.[12] This chapter describes results using SS-OCT at 400,000 A-scans per second, factors of 4–5 times faster than current commercial OCT technology.

PRINCIPLES OF OCTA

As described in previous chapters, OCTA generates three dimensional images of vascular structure without requiring the injection of exogenous dyes, such as fluorescein or indocyanine green. OCTA imaging protocols acquire multiple cross sectional images (B-scans) from the same retinal position in order to detect changes that are produced by flowing erythrocytes. If the tissue is stationary, then all of the pixels in repeated B-scans will be the same. However, if there is motion from blood flow there will be fluctuations in the OCT intensity or phase. These fluctuations can be characterized by a decorrelation signal which is calculated at each pixel. A number of techniques for OCTA using intensity and/or phase information have been previously described.[13-21]

SS-OCTA OF THE RETINAL VASCULATURE IN NORMAL EYES

Figure 21.2, which shows an example of structural OCT and OCTA of a normal retina, illustrates the importance of ultrahigh speed in achieving wide field imaging. The images were obtained using prototype SS-OCT technology with a vertical cavity surface emitting laser (VCSEL) light source at 400,000 A-scans per second with a 9.6 um axial resolution at 1,060 nm. OCTA was performed by repeatedly acquiring 5 B-scans from the same retinal position, each consisting of 500 A-scans with 500 different B-scan positions in the volumetric data set. Each OCTA data set required 500 × 5 × 500 A-scans and was acquired in ~3.9 seconds. The figure shows *en face* OCTA over different fields of view, ranging from 12 mm × 12 mm to 3 mm × 3 mm. Note that each field of

view differs by a factor of 2 in linear dimension or a factor of 4 in area. If future OCT instruments operate at 200,000 to 400,000 A-scans per second, ~2 to 4 times faster than current instruments, they will enable a ~1.4 to 2 times larger linear field to be imaged while maintaining the same resolution.

SS-OCTA OF THE CHORIOCAPILLARIS VASCULATURE IN NORMAL EYES

Since OCTA generates three dimensional images of vasculature, both retinal and choroidal vascular structure can be obtained from the same data set. Imaging the choroid and choriocapillaris, the capillary network of the choroid, is important as much as alterations in choroidal and choriocapillaris vasculature may serve as early markers for several retinal diseases. In particular, choroidal circulation supplies oxygen to the outer retinal layers, and alterations in the choroid/choriocapillaris are associated with posterior segment diseases such as age-related macular degeneration (AMD) and diabetic retinopathy (DR).[22-24] Imaging the choriocapillaris is especially challenging because it is located behind the pigmented RPE, is quite thin, even in healthy eyes, and has a dense lobular microvasculature that requires high pixel densities to resolve. A number of previous studies using *en face* structural OCT have investigated the choriocapillaris. Motaghiannezam et al. demonstrated visualization of the choriocapillaris and larger choroidal vessels in the Sattler's

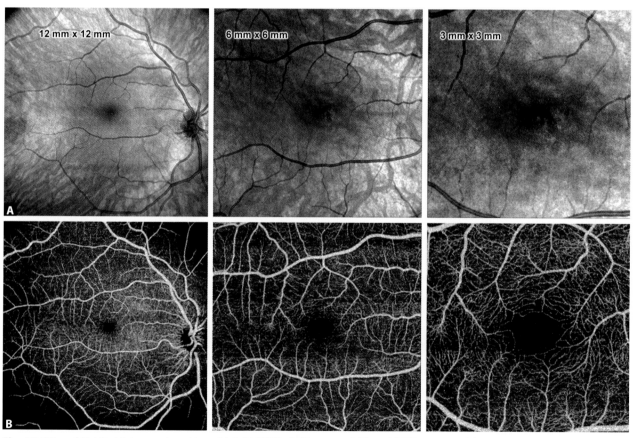

Figs 21.2A and B: Ultrahigh speed enables widefield OCTA. OCT structural (A) and OCTA images of the retina (B). As the scanning area is reduced from 12 mm x 12 mm to 3 mm x 3 mm, there is an increase in the A-scan density per fundus area, which allows finer vascular detail to be visualized.

and Haller's layers in normal subjects using SS-OCT at the 57,000 A-scans per second.[25] Sohrab et al. also studied the choriocapillaris and larger choroidal vessel patterns with SD-OCT in patients with early AMD or reticular pseudo-drusen.[26] While structural OCT of the choriocapillaris can be clinically useful, OCTA can be more sensitive for visualizing alterations in vascular structure.

OCTA of the choriocapillaris in normal subjects was demonstrated using adaptive optics and Doppler phase techniques with long wavelength SD-OCT at 91,000 A-scans per second by Kurokawa et al. in 2012.[27] OCTA of the choriocapillaris in a normal subject was also demonstrated using long wavelength SS-OCT at 100,000 A-scans per second combined with SLO eye tracking by Braaf et al. in 2013.[28] Studies in an AMD patient and a normal subject were reported by Kim et al. in 2013 using phase variance OCTA of the choriocapillaris with SD-OCT.[29] These studies were all performed with acquisition speeds of ~100,000 A-scans per second and used relatively long imaging times or small fields of view.

Figure 21.3 shows *en face* OCT intensity and OCTA images of the choriocapillaris of a normal subject generated by mosaicking smaller 3 mm × 3 mm fields over a 32 mm field spanning the macula and peripheral retina from Choi et al.[30] Small fields of view were acquired over a wide span in order to compare OCTA images with the morphology of the choriocapillaris across the fundus. Imaging was performed using a prototype SS-OCT instrument using a VCSEL light source operating at 400,000 A-scans per second with a 9.6 um axial resolution at 1,060 nm. OCTA was performed by repeatedly acquiring 4 B-scans from the same retinal position, each consisting of 800 A-scans with

400 different B-scan positions in the volumetric data set. Each OCTA data set required 800 × 4 × 400 A-scans and was acquired in 3.8 seconds. The *en face* OCTA images of Figure 21.3 agree with known histological and electron micrograph corrosion casting studies, which have shown that the capillary density and pattern in the choriocapillaris are a function of the fundus location. In particular, the choriocapillaris has a densely-packed honeycomb structure at the central fovea, and a more lobular and less dense structure towards the equator and periphery.[31-34]

SS-OCTA IN PATIENTS WITH DIABETES

OCTA is a powerful technique for visualizing alterations that occur in diseases of the retinal vasculature, such as in diabetic retinopathy. Figure 21.4A compares fundus photography, fluorescein angiography (FA), and ultrahigh speed SS-OCTA of a 45-year-old male patient with diabetic retinopathy. The fluorescein angiogram exhibits multiple small microaneurysms Fig. 21.4B, vascular remodeling, and enlargement of the foveal avascular zone. It is important to note that OCTA visualizes flow and therefore microaneurysms and capillaries with slow flow may appear silent on OCTA. Most microvascular features are visualized at least as well and possibly better in the OCTA image of the retinal vasculature, which shows vascular pruning and remodeling, enlargement and irregularity of the foveal avascular zone, and capillary dropout, especially temporal to the foveal avascular zone. The additional advantage of OCTA is that because fluorescein is not required, the imaging results from the 'acute' eye are the same as 'late' or 'intermediate' eye; OCTA of both eyes can be performed with equal detail. Figure 21.4C shows an OCTA image of the contralateral eye.

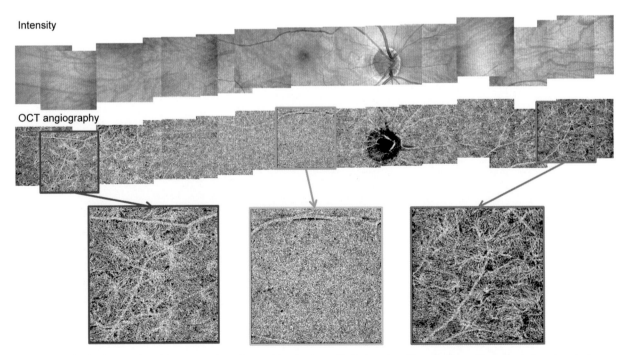

Fig. 21.3: Ultrahigh speed and long wavelengths enable choriocapillaris imaging. The choriocapillaris is challenging to image because of its fine vascular structure and its location below the RPE. This example shows mosaic imaging with small regions at various fundus locations from the macula to the periphery. *Note* the lobular organization of the choriocapillaris vasculature in the periphery which becomes finer in the macular region, consistent with known morphology. (*Adapted* from: Choi et al. Plos One, 2013)

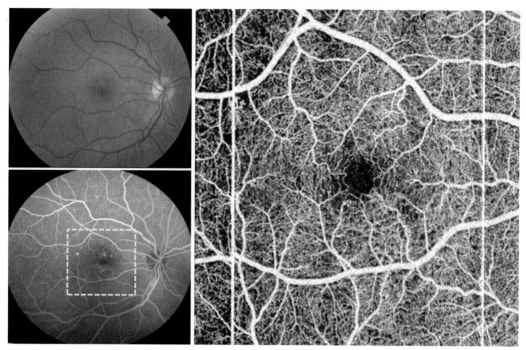

Fig. 21.4A: Moderate NPDR with DME. OCTA of a 45-year-old man with moderate nonproliferative diabetic retinopathy and diabetic macular edema. *Note* the retinal vascular detail visible on the OCTA image on the right.

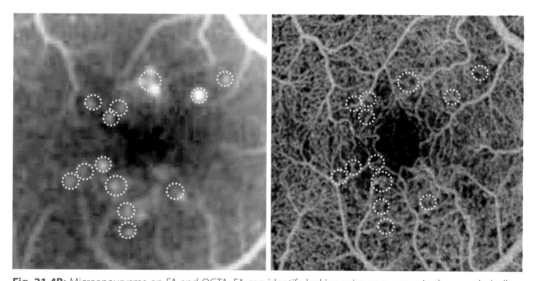

Fig. 21.4B: Microaneurysms on FA and OCTA. FA can identify leaking microaneurysms in the macula (yellow circles). OCTA shows that most of the leaking microaneurysms are located adjacent to areas of capillary nonperfusion, a detail that cannot be appreciated in the FA. Moreover, OCTA also identifies nonleaking aneurysms (examples outlined with red circles).

OCTA has the limitation that it cannot visualize alterations in vascular permeability, whereas FA shows dye leakage from abnormal retinal blood vessels. However, hyperfluorescence from dye leakage in FA can also be a disadvantage because it can obscure fine vascular structure. In addition, since structural OCT images are acquired simultaneously with OCTA, a retinal thickness map that is precisely registered to the OCTA volume can be generated, and areas of retinal thickening can be used as a surrogate for leakage. When coupled with the ability to visualize microaneurysms on OCTA, structural OCT thickness maps can

be a useful guide for application of focal laser, one of the most important clinical indications for mapping fluorescein dye leakage.

In addition, simultaneous choriocapillaris OCTA images can also be obtained on diabetic patients. Figure 21.5 shows an OCTA images from a 68-year-old male patient with a history of non-insulin dependent diabetes mellitus without clinically evident diabetic retinopathy, exhibiting patchy loss or reduction in flow in the choriocapillaris. Our studies indicate that patchy or diffuse loss or flow reduction in the choriocapillaris is present

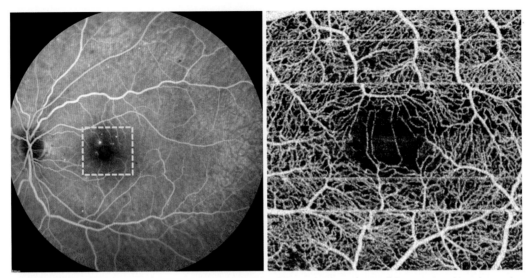

Fig. 21.4C: FA and OCTA of the contralateral eye. OCTA of the contralateral eye of the same patient shows the same level of detail as visualized in the right eye. Since OCTA does not require dye, there is no 'acute' and 'late' eye on the OCTA image. Vasculature in both eyes can be visualized in equal detail.

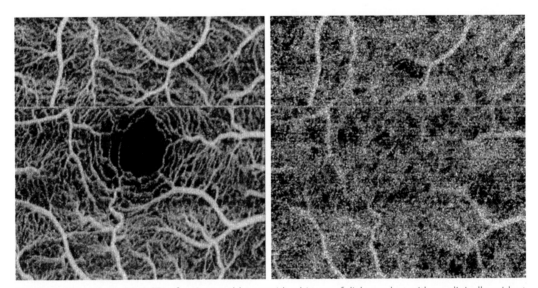

Fig. 21.5: DM without DR. OCTA of a 68-year-old man with a history of diabetes, but with no clinically evident diabetic retinopathy. OCTA shows normal retinal vasculature, but patchy atrophy or flow impairment in the choriocapillaris.

in many patients with diabetes, even in the absence of diabetic retinopathy. This correlates with histopathologic observations made in the eyes of diabetics with no clinical evidence of diabetic retinopathy.[24]

SS-OCTA IN PATIENTS WITH NON-EXUDATIVE AMD

SS-OCTA promises to be especially useful in studying non-exudative age-related macular degeneration (AMD), where the choroidal/choriocapillaris vasculature is suspected to play an important role in disease pathogenesis. Fluorescein angiography (FA) and indocyanine angiography (ICGA) are not well-suited to imaging the choriocapillaris, due to leakage, attenuation of the

excitation wavelengths by the RPE, and an inability to perform depth resolved imaging. In contrast, OCTA using long wavelength, ultrahigh speed SS-OCT enables detailed visualization of the choriocapillaris. Taken together with structural OCT volumes, OCTA data may enable researchers to identify structural or flow markers that predict progression of macular degeneration, as well as to better understand the pathogenesis of disease.

Figure 21.6 shows OCT and OCTA images from a 68, a 79, and an 87-year-old patient, all with non-exudative AMD without geographic atrophy (GA). These images are organized according to severity of pathology. The alteration of the choriocapillaris shown in the second row is greater than that in the first row, and similarly with the third and second rows. *Note* that the alteration of the RPE/inner segment (IS)/outer segment (OS)

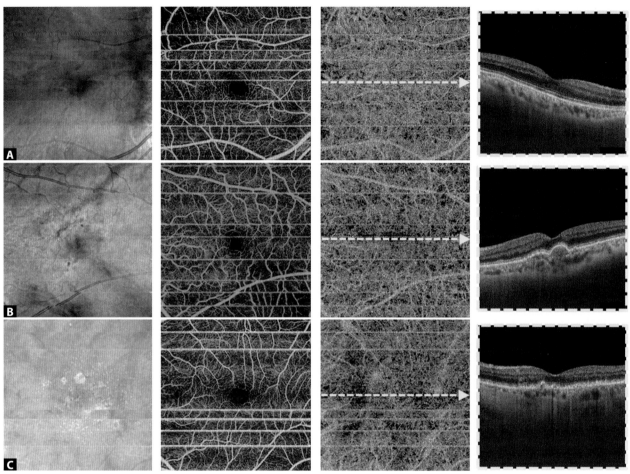

Figs 21.6A to C: Non-exudative AMD without GA. OCT and OCTA images from a 68 (first row), a 79 (second row), and an 87 (third row) year old patient, all with non-exudative AMD without GA. The first column shows OCT projections through the entire volume; the second column shows OCTA projections through the depths spanned by the retinal vasculature; the third column shows slabs from the OCTA volume taken at the depth of the choriocapillaris; the fourth column shows OCT B-scans extracted at the position of the yellow arrows. Note that the severity of choriocapillaris alteration follows the same trend as the severity RPE/IS/OS alteration.

layers in the corresponding cross-sectional B-scans follows the same trend. We have observed that, in general, eyes with more severe choriocapillaris alteration have more severe alteration of the RPE/IS/OS layers. However, in cases of non-exudative AMD without GA, we did not observe an obvious spatial association between areas of CC alteration and areas of RPE/IS/OS alteration.

Figure 21.7 shows OCT and OCTA images from a 78-year-old patient with a history of GA, secondary to AMD. The *en face* OCTA of the choriocapillaris slab shows choriocapillaris atrophy in the region of GA, which is indicated by the dashed red contour. Choriocapillaris alteration beyond the boundaries of GA is also apparent. In our SS-OCTA studies, we have observed choriocapillaris atrophy within the region of GA, and in some—but not all—patients, choriocapillaris alteration was observed beyond the boundaries of GA.

For OCTA imaging of the choriocapillaris, the longer 1,050 nm wavelengths used in SS-OCTA systems provides a significant advantage compared to the shorter 840 nm wavelengths used in SD-OCTA systems. The primary reason for this advantage is that 840 nm light is absorbed by the RPE and deposits, such as drusen. In comparison, longer wavelength 1,050 nm light is less

strongly absorbed. In general, areas of low OCT signal cannot be used to generate reliable OCTA images. OCTA protocols typically remove or mask out areas with low OCT structural signals, which in turn cause these area to appear to have no flow in OCTA images. Figure 21.8 illustrates the difference between 840 nm SD-OCTA and 1,050 nm SS-OCTA images of the choriocapillaris taken from the same 74-year-old patient with non-exudative AMD. The first and second rows show OCT and OCTA images acquired from an SD-OCTA system (Optovue Inc.) and a prototype SS-OCTA system, respectively. The red arrow in the SD-OCT slab indicates a region of low signal underlying a druse; the red arrow in the corresponding SD-OCTA slab appears to show choriocapillaris alteration. However, the SS-OCTA image in the third column shows that the choriocapillaris is intact and that the apparent choriocapillaris alteration in the SD-OCTA image is an artifact introduced by low signal levels. The yellow arrows in the SS-OCTA image point to an artifact caused by a segmentation error, where the OCTA slab position is incorrect and does not span the choriocapillaris. This example suggests that structural and angiographic images should be reviewed in a coordinated manner to reduce the potential of misinterpretation.

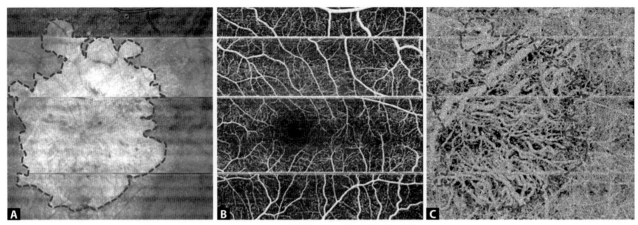

Fig. 21.7A to C: Non-exudative AMD with GA. OCTA in a 78-year-old patient with a history of GA, secondary to AMD. (A) It shows a projection of the OCT volume with the region of GA demarcated by a yellow contour. (B) This image shows a projection of the OCTA volume through the depths spanned by the retinal vasculature. (C) This shows a slab of the OCTA volume taken at the depth of the choriocapillaris.

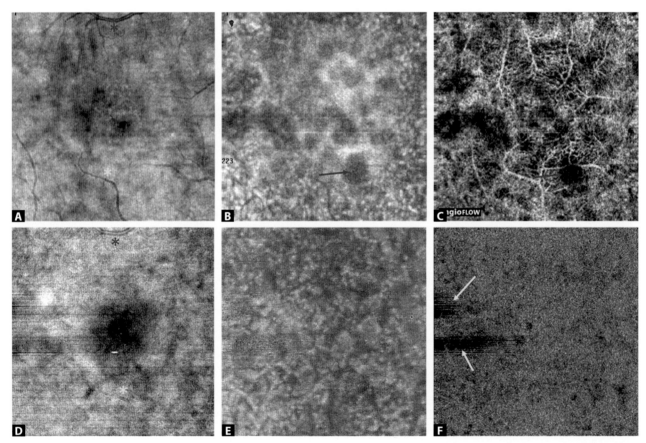

Figs 21.8A to F: SD-OCTA and SS-OCTA imaging of choriocapillaris under drusen. SD-OCTA (A to C) and SS-OCTA (D to F) images of the choriocapillaris in the same 74-year-old patient with non-exudative AMD. Fundus projections of the OCT volume are shown in the first column; the correspondence of the retinal vasculature (*) between the SD-OCT and SS-OCT images establishes that the two fields of view are nearly identical. OCT slabs (B, E) and OCTA slabs (C, F) are both taken at the level of the choriocapillaris. Low signal under a drusen, indicated by the red arrow, introduces an artifact into the SD-OCTA image that makes it appear as though there is no flow (artifactual choriocapillaris alteration) under the druse. The SS-OCTA image does not suffer from the same artifact. Yellow arrows point to a segmentation error.

SUMMARY

OCTA is a powerful, noninvasive method for visualizing retinal and choroidal vasculature. As OCTA becomes more widely available, and as comprehensive clinical information emerges, it promises to have a significant impact on the understanding disease pathogenesis, on pharmaceutical development, and on clinical practice. Next generation SS-OCT technology promises to enable widefield OCTA that provides, simultaneously, detailed images of the retinal and choriocapillaris vasculatures. Furthermore, the longer wavelength of SS-OCTA systems enables superior imaging of the choriocapillaris compared to SD-OCTA systems. Since OCTA images are prone to artifacts, they require more careful clinical interpretation than OCT structural images. More detailed clinical studies are required in order to identify specific indications for OCTA as well as diagnostic criteria and surrogate markers of disease. However continuing advances in OCT technology promise to improve OCTA performance and enable wider clinical utility.

ACKNOWLEDGMENTS

The authors gratefully acknowledge Mehreen Adhi and Tarek Alasil for assistance with imaging; ByungKun Lee, Chen Lu, and Jonathan Liu for developing the swept source technology; Benjamin Potsaid and Alex Cable from Thorlabs; Vijaysekhar Jayaraman from Praevium Research for developing VCSEL laser technology. We also gratefully acknowledge support from the National Institute of Health (NIH R01-EY011289-27, R44-EY022864-01, R44-EY022864-02, R01-CA075289-16), Air Force Office of Scientific Research (AFOSR FA9550-10-1-0551 and FA9550-12-1-0499), a Samsung Scholarship, and by a Natural Sciences and Engineering Research Council of Canada Scholarship.

REFERENCES

1. Golubovic B, Bouma BE, Tearney GJ, Fujimoto JG. Optical frequency-domain reflectometry using rapid wavelength tuning of a Cr4+: Forsterite laser. Opt Lett. 1997;22(22):1704-6.

2. Chinn SR, Swanson EA, Fujimoto JG. Optical coherence tomography using a frequency-tunable optical source. Opt Lett. 1997;22(5):340-2.

3. Unterhuber A, Povazay B, Hermann B, Sattmann H, Chavez-Pirson A, Drexler W. In vivo retinal optical coherence tomography at 1040 nm-enhanced penetration into the choroid. Optics Express. 2005;13(9): 3252-8.

4. Povazay B, Hermann B, Unterhuber A, Hofer B, Sattmann H, Zeiler F, et al. Three-dimensional optical coherence tomography at 1050 nm versus 800 nm in retinal pathologies: Enhanced performance and choroidal penetration in cataract patients. J Biomed Opt. 2007;12(4).

5. Yun SH, Tearney GJ, Bouma BE, Park BH, de Boer JF. High-speed spectral-domain optical coherence tomography at 1.3 mu m wavelength. Optics Express. 2003;11(26):3598-604.

6. Oh WY, Yun SH, Tearney GJ, Bouma BE. 115 kHz tuning repetition rate ultrahigh-speed wavelength-swept semiconductor laser. Opt Lett. 2005;30(23):3159-61.

7. Huber R, Wojtkowski M, Fujimoto JG. Fourier Domain Mode Locking (FDML): A new laser operating regime and applications for optical coherence tomography. Optics Express. 2006;14(8):3225-37.

8. Srinivasan VJ, Monson BK, Wojtkowski M, Bilonick RA, Gorczynska I, Chen R, et al. Characterization of outer retinal morphology with high-speed, ultrahigh-resolution optical coherence tomography. Invest Ophthalmol Vis Sci. 2008;49(4):1571-9.

9. Klein T, Wieser W, Eigenwillig CM, Biedermann BR, Huber R. Megahertz OCT for ultrawide-field retinal imaging with a 1050 nm Fourier domain mode-locked laser. Optics Express. 2011;19(4):3044-62.

10. Yasuno Y, Hong YJ, Makita S, Yamanari M, Akiba M, Miura M, et al. In vivo high-contrast imaging of deep posterior eye by 1-mu m swept source optical coherence tomography and scattering optical coherence angiography. Optics Express. 2007;15(10):6121-39.

11. Potsaid B, Baumann B, Huang D, Barry S, Cable AE, Schuman JS, et al. Ultrahigh speed 1050nm swept source/Fourier domain OCT retinal and anterior segment imaging at 100,000 to 400,000 axial scans per second. Optics Express. 2010;18(19):20029-48.

12. Grulkowski I, Liu JJ, Potsaid B, Jayaraman V, Lu CD, Jiang J, et al. Retinal, anterior segment and full eye imaging using ultrahigh speed swept source OCT with vertical-cavity surface emitting lasers. Biomedical optics express. 2012;3(11):2733-51.

13. Makita S, Hong Y, Yamanari M, Yatagai T, Yasuno Y. Optical coherence angiography. Optics Express. 2006;14(17):7821-40.

14. Fingler J, Schwartz D, Yang CH, Fraser SE. Mobility and transverse flow visualization using phase variance contrast with spectral domain optical coherence tomography. Optics Express. 2007;15(20):12636-53.

15. Tao YK, Kennedy KM, Izatt JA. Velocity-resolved 3D retinal microvessel imaging using single-pass flow imaging spectral domain optical coherence tomography. Optics Express. 2009;17(5):4177-88.

16. An L, Wang RKK. In vivo volumetric imaging of vascular perfusion within human retina and choroids with optical micro-angiography. Optics Express. 2008;16(15):11438-52.

17. Mariampillai A, Standish BA, Moriyama EH, Khurana M, Munce NR, Leung MKK, et al. Speckle variance detection of microvasculature using swept-source optical coherence tomography. Opt Lett. 2008;33(13):1530-2.

18. Vakoc BJ, Lanning RM, Tyrrell JA, Padera TP, Bartlett LA, Stylianopoulos T, et al. Three-dimensional microscopy of the tumor microenvironment in vivo using optical frequency domain imaging. Nat Med. 2009;15(10): 1219-U151.

19. Yu LF, Chen ZP. Doppler variance imaging for three-dimensional retina and choroid angiography. J Biomed Opt. 2010;15(1).

20. Enfield J, Jonathan E, Leahy M. In vivo imaging of the microcirculation of the volar forearm using correlation mapping optical coherence tomography (cmOCT). Biomedical Optics Express. 2011;2(5):1184-93.

21. Blatter C, Klein T, Grajciar B, Schmoll T, Wieser W, Andre R, et al. Ultrahigh-speed non-invasive widefield angiography. J Biomed Opt. 2012;17(7).

22. Schmetterer L, Kiel J. Ocular Blood Flow. Berlin, Heidelberg: Springer; 2012.

23. Lutty GA, Cao JT, McLeod DS. Relationship of polymorphonuclear leukocytes to capillary dropout in the human diabetic choroid. Am J Pathol. 1997;151(3):707-14.

24. Cao JT, McLeod DS, Merges CA, Lutty GA. Choriocapillaris degeneration and related pathologic changes in human diabetic eyes. Archives of Ophthalmology. 1998;116(5):589-97.

25. Motaghiannezam R, Schwartz DM, Fraser SE. In vivo human choroidal vascular pattern visualization using high-speed swept-source optical coherence tomography at 1060 nm. Invest Ophthalmo Visual Science. 2012;53(4):2337-48.

26. Sohrab M, Wu K, Fawzi AA. A Pilot study of morphometric analysis of choroidal vasculature in vivo, using en face optical coherence tomography. Plos One. 2012;7(11).

27. Kurokawa K, Sasaki K, Makita S, Hong YJ, Yasuno Y. Three-dimensional retinal and choroidal capillary imaging by power Doppler optical coherence angiography with adaptive optics. Optics Express. 2012;20(20):22796-812. Epub 2012/10/06.

28. Braaf B, Vienola KV, Sheehy CK, Yang Q, Vermeer KA, Tiruveedhula P, et al. Real-time eye motion correction in phase-resolved OCT angiography with tracking SLO. Biomedical Optics Express. 2013;4(1):51-65.

29. Kim DY, Fingler J, Zawadzki RJ, Park SS, Morse LS, Schwartz DM, et al. Optical imaging of the chorioretinal vasculature in the living human eye. Proc Natl Acad Sci U S A. 2013;110(35):14354-9.

30. Choi W, Mohler KJ, Potsaid B, Lu CD, Liu JJ, Jayaraman V, et al. Choriocapillaris and choroidal microvasculature imaging with ultrahigh speed OCT angiography. Plos One. 2013;8(12).

31. Yoneya S, Tso MOM. Angioarchitecture of the human choroid. Archives of Ophthalmology. 1987;105(5):681-7.

32. Olver JM. Functional-anatomy of the choroidal circulation—Methyl-methacrylate casting of human choroid. Eye. 1990;4:262-72.

33. Mcleod DS, Lutty GA. High-resolution histological analysis of the human choroidal vasculature. Invest Ophthalmo & Vis Sci. 1994;35(4):3799-811.

34. Zhang HR. Scanning electron-microscopic study of corrosion casts on retinal and choroidal angioarchitecture in man and animals. Progress in setinal Eye Res. 1994;13(1):243-70.

Index

Page numbers followed by '*f*' and '*t*' indicate figures and tables respectively.